the fast diet

the
fast
diet

DR MICHAEL MOSLEY
& MIMI SPENCER

All photographs by Romas Foord

Published in 2013 by Short Books
3A Exmouth House
Pine Street
EC1R 0JH

14

A CIP catalogue record for this book
is available from the British Library.

ISBN 978-1-78072-167-5

Printed in Great Britain by CPI Group (UK) Ltd. Croydon, CR0 4YY

For my wife Clare and children Alex, Jack, Daniel and
Kate – who make living longer worthwhile. *MM*

———————

For Ned, Lily May and Paul – my Brighton rock. And for
my parents, who have always known that food is love. *MS*

CONTENTS

INTRODUCTION

Over the last few decades, food fads have come and gone, but the standard medical advice on what constitutes a healthy lifestyle has stayed much the same: eat low-fat foods, exercise more... and never, ever skip meals. Over that same period, levels of obesity worldwide have soared.

So is there a different, evidence-based approach? One that relies on science, not opinion? Well, we think there is. Intermittent Fasting.

When we first read about the alleged benefits of Intermittent Fasting, we, like many, were sceptical. Fasting seemed drastic, difficult – and we both knew that dieting, of any description, is generally doomed to fail. But now that we've looked at it in depth and tried it ourselves, we are convinced of its remarkable potential. As one of the medical experts interviewed for this book puts it: 'There is nothing else you can do to your body that is as powerful as fasting.'

Fasting: an ancient idea, a modern method

Fasting is nothing new. As we'll discover in the next chapter, your body is designed to fast. We evolved at a time when food was scarce; we are the product of millennia of feast and famine. The reason we respond so well to Intermittent Fasting is that it mimics, far more accurately than three meals a day, the environment in which modern humans were shaped.

Fasting, of course, remains an article of faith for many. The fasts of Lent, Yom Kippur and Ramadan are just some of the better-known examples. Greek Orthodox Christians are encouraged to fast for 180 days of the year (according to Saint Nikolai of Zicha, 'Gluttony makes a man gloomy and fearful, but fasting makes him joyful and courageous'), while Buddhist monks fast on the new moon and full moon of each lunar month.

Many more of us, however, seem to be eating most of the time. We're rarely ever hungry. But we are dissatisfied. With our weight, our bodies, our health.

Intermittent Fasting can put us back in touch with our human selves. It is a route not only to weight loss, but also to long-term health and wellbeing. Scientists are only just beginning to discover and prove how powerful a tool it can be.

This book is a product of that cutting-edge research and its impact on our current thinking about weight loss, disease resistance and longevity. But it is also the result of our personal experience. Both are relevant here – the lab and the lifestyle – so we investigate Intermittent Fasting from two complementary perspectives. First, Michael, who used his body and medical training to test its potential, explains the scientific foundations of Intermittent Fasting and the 5:2 diet – something he brought to the world's attention last summer.

Then Mimi offers a practical guide on how to do it safely, effectively and in a sustainable way, a way that will fit easily into your normal, everyday life. She looks in detail at how fasting feels, what you can expect from day to day, what to eat and when to eat – and provides a host of tips and strategies to help you gain the greatest benefit from the diet's simple precepts.

As you'll see below, the Fast Diet has changed both of our lives. We hope it will do the same for you.

Michael's motivation: a male perspective

I am a 55-year-old male and before I embarked on my exploration of Intermittent Fasting I was mildly overweight: at 5'11", I weighed around 85kg (13 stone 6lb) and had a Body Mass Index ((BMI) of 26, which put me into the overweight category. Until my mid-30s, I had been slim, but like many people I then gradually put on weight, around 0.5kg a year. This doesn't sound much, but over a couple of decades it pushed me up and up.

Slowly I realised that I was starting to resemble my father, a man who struggled with his weight all his life and died in his early 70s of complications associated with diabetes. At his funeral many of his friends commented on how like him I had become.

I was fortunate enough, while making a documentary for the BBC, to have an MRI scan done. This revealed that I am a TOFI, Thin on the Outside and Fat Inside. This is the most dangerous sort of fat, visceral fat, because it wraps itself around your internal organs and puts you at risk of heart disease and diabetes. I later had blood tests that showed I was heading towards diabetes, with a cholesterol score that was also way too high. Clearly I was going to have to do something about this. I tried following standard advice. Except it made little difference. My weight and blood profile remained stuck in the 'danger ahead' zone.

I had never tried dieting before because I'd never found a diet that I thought would work. I watched my father try every form of diet, from Scarsdale through Atkins, from the Cambridge Diet to the Drinking Man's Diet. He lost weight on each one of them, and then within a few months put it all back on, and more.

Then, at the beginning of 2012, I was approached by Aidan Laverty, editor of the BBC science series *Horizon*, who asked if I would like to put myself forward as a guinea pig to explore the science behind life extension. I wasn't sure what we would find, but, along with producer Kate

Dart and researcher Roshan Samarasinghe, we quickly focused on calorie restriction and fasting as a fruitful area to explore.

Calorie restriction (CR) is pretty brutal; it involves eating an awful lot less than a normal person would expect to eat, and doing so every day of your – hopefully – long life The reason people put themselves through this is that it is the only intervention that has been shown to extend lifespan, at least in animals. There are around 50,000 CHRONies (Calorie Restrictors on Optimal Nutrition) worldwide, and I have met quite a number of them. Despite their generally fabulous biochemical profile, I have never been seriously tempted to join their skinny ranks. I simply don't have the will-power or desire to live permanently on an extreme low-calorie diet.

So I was delighted to discover Intermittent Fasting (IF), which involves eating fewer calories, but only some of the time. If the science was right, it offered the benefits of CR, but without the pain.

I set off around the US, meeting leading scientists who generously shared their research and ideas with me. It became clear that IF was no fad. But it wouldn't be as easy as I'd originally hoped. As you'll see later in the book, there are many different forms of Intermittent Fasting. Some involve eating nothing for 24 hours or longer. Others involve a single, low-calorie meal once a day, every other day. I tried both but couldn't imagine doing either on a regular basis. I found it was simply too hard.

Instead I decided to create and test my own, modified version. Five days a week, I would eat normally; on the remaining two I would eat a quarter of my usual calorie intake (i.e. 600 calories).

I split the 600 calories in two – around 250 calories for breakfast and 350 calories for supper – effectively fasting for 12 hours at a stretch. I also decided to split my fasting days: I would fast on Mondays and Thursdays. I became my own experiment.

The programme, *Eat, Fast, Live Longer*, which detailed my adventures with what we were now calling the 5:2 diet, went out on the BBC during the London Olympics in August 2012. I expected it to be lost in the media frenzy that surrounded the Games, but instead it generated a frenzy of its own. The programme was watched by over 2.5 million people – a huge audience for *Horizon* – and hundreds of thousands more on YouTube. My Twitter account, @DrMichaelMosley, went into overdrive, my followers tripled; everyone wanted to try my version of Intermittent Fasting and they were all asking me what they should do.

The newspapers took up the story. Articles appeared in *The Times*, *The Daily Telegraph*, *The Daily Mail* and *The Mail on Sunday*. Before long, it was picked up by newspapers all over the world – in New York, Los Angeles, Paris, Madrid, Montreal, Islamabad and Delhi. Online groups were created, menus and experiences swapped, chat rooms started buzzing about fasting.

People began to stop me on the street and tell me how well they were doing on the 5:2 diet. They also emailed details of their experiences. Among those emails, a surprisingly large number were from doctors. Like me, they had initially been sceptical, but they had tried it for themselves, found that it worked and had begun suggesting it to their patients. They wanted information, menus, details of the scientific research to scrutinise. They wanted me to write a book. I hedged, procrastinated, then finally found a collaborator, Mimi Spencer, whom I liked and trusted and who has an in-depth knowledge of food. Which is how what you are reading came about.

Michael's background

I trained as a doctor at the Royal Free Hospital in London and after qualifying joined the BBC as a trainee assistant producer. Over the last 25 years I have made numerous science and history documentaries for the BBC, first behind the camera, more recently as a presenter. I was executive producer of *QED*, *Trust Me I'm a Doctor* and *Superhuman*. I worked with John Cleese, Jeremy Clarkson, Professor Robert Winston, Sir David Attenborough and Professor Alice Roberts. I devised and executive-produced three of the most popular science or history programmes of the last decade: *Pompeii – the last day*, *Supervolcano* and *Krakatoa*.

As a presenter I have made a dozen series for the BBC, including *Medical Mavericks*, *Blood and Guts*, *Inside Michael Mosley*, *Science Story*, *The Young Ones*, *Inside the Human Body* and *The Truth about Exercise*. I am currently making three new series, as well as being a regular science presenter for the BBC's *One Show*.

I have won numerous awards, including being named Medical Journalist of the Year by the British Medical Association.

Mimi's motivation: a female perspective

I started Intermittent Fasting on the day I was commissioned to write a feature for *The Times* about Michael's *Horizon* programme. It was the first I'd heard of Intermittent Fasting, and the idea appealed immediately, even to a cynical soul who has spent two decades examining the curious acrobatics of the fashion industry, the beauty business and the diet trade.

I'd dabbled in diets before – show me a 40-something woman who hasn't – losing weight, then losing faith within weeks and piling it all back on. Though never overweight, I'd long been interested in dropping that reluctant half a stone or more – the pounds I picked up in pregnancy and somehow never lost. The diets I tried were always too hard to follow, too complicated to implement, too boring, too tough, too single-strand, too invasive, sucking the juice out of life and leaving you with the scraps. There was nothing I found that I could adopt and thread into the context of my life – as a mother, a working woman, a wife.

I've argued for years that dieting is a fool's game, doomed to fail because of the restrictions and deprivations imposed on an otherwise happy life, but this felt immediately different. The scientific evidence was extensive and compelling, and (crucially for me) the medical community was positive. The effects, for Michael and others, were impressive, startling even. In his *Horizon* documentary, Michael called it 'the beginning of something huge... which could radically transform the nation's health'. I couldn't resist. Nor could I conceive of a reason to wait.

In the months since I wrote *The Times* feature, I have remained a convert. An evangelist, actually. I'm still 'on' the Fast Diet now, but I barely notice it. At the outset, I weighed 60kg (around nine and a half stone). At 5'7", my BMI was an OK 21.4. Today, as I write, I weigh 54kg (eight and a half stone) with a BMI of 19.4. That's a weight off. I feel light, lean and alive. Fasting has become part of my weekly life, something I do automatically without stressing about it.

Six months in, I have more energy, more bounce, clearer skin, a greater zest for life. And, it has to be said, new jeans (27-inch waist) and none of my annual bikini dread as summer approaches. But, perhaps more importantly, I know that there's a long-term gain. I'm doing the best for my body and my brain. It's an intimate revelation, but one worth sharing.

Mimi's background

I have written about fashion, food and body shape in national newspapers and magazines for 20 years, starting out at *Vogue*, followed by *The Guardian*, *The Observer* and *The London Evening Standard*, where I was named British Fashion Journalist of the Year in 2000. I am currently a columnist for the *Mail on Sunday*'s *You Magazine* and a regular features writer for *The Saturday Times*. In 2009, I wrote a book, *101 Things to Do Before you Diet*, cataloguing my dismay with fad regimes, and their hopeless yo-yo of loss and gain. Intermittent Fasting is the only plan I have discovered in two decades that gets the weight off and keeps it off. And the anti-ageing health benefits? Gravy.

The Fast Diet: the potential, the promise

We know that for many people the standard diet advice simply does not work. The Fast Diet is a radical alternative. It has the potential to change the way we think about eating and weight loss.

- The Fast Diet demands we think not just about what we eat, but when we eat it

- There are no complicated rules to follow; the strategy is flexible, comprehensible and user-friendly

- There is no daily slog of calorie control – none of the boredom, frustration or serial deprivation that characterise conventional diet plans

- Yes, it involves fasting, but not as you know it; you won't 'starve' on any given day

- You will still enjoy the foods you love. Most of the time

- Once the weight is off, sticking to the basic programme will mean that it stays off

- Weight loss is only one benefit of the Fast Diet. The real dividend is the potential long-term health gains, cutting your risk of a range of diseases, including diabetes, heart disease and cancer

- You will soon come to understand that it is not just a diet. It is much more than that: it is a sustainable strategy for a healthy, long life

Now, you'll want to understand exactly how we can make these dramatic assertions. In the next chapter, Michael explains the science that makes the Fast Diet tick.

THE SCIENCE OF FASTING

For most animals out in the wild, periods of feast and famine are the norm. Our remote ancestors did not often eat four or five meals a day. Instead they would kill, gorge, lie around and then have to go for long periods of time without having anything to eat. Our bodies and our genes were forged in an environment of scarcity, punctuated by the occasional massive blow-out.

These days, of course, things are very different. We eat all the time. Fasting – the voluntary abstaining from eating food – is seen as a rather eccentric, not to mention unhealthy, thing to do. Most of us expect to eat at least three meals a day and have substantial snacks in between. In addition to the meals and the snacks, we also graze; a milky cappuccino here, the odd biscuit there, or maybe a smoothie because it's 'healthier'.

Once upon a time parents told their children not to eat between meals. Those times are long gone. Recent research in the US, which compared the eating habits of 28,000 children and 36,000 adults over the last thirty years, found that the amount of time spent between what the researchers coyly described as 'eating occasions' has fallen by an average of an hour. In other words, over the last few decades the amount of time we spend 'not eating' has dropped dramatically.[1] In the 1970s, people like my mother would go around four and a half hours without eating, while children like me would be expected to last about four hours between meals. Now it's down to three and a half hours for adults and three hours for children, and that doesn't include all the drinks and nibbles.

The idea that eating little and often is a 'good thing' has partly been driven by snack manufacturers and faddish diet books, but it has also had support from the medical establishment. Their argument is that it is better to eat lots of small meals because that way we are less likely to get hungry and gorge on high-fat junk. I can appreciate the argument, and there have been some studies that suggest there are health benefits to eating small meals regularly, as long as you don't simply end up eating more. Unfortunately, in the real world that's exactly what happens.

In the study I quoted above, they found that compared to 30 years ago, we not only eat around 180 calories a day more in snacks – much of it in the form of milky and fizzey drinks and smoothies – but we also eat more when it comes to our regular meals, up by an average of 120 calories a day.

In other words, snacking doesn't seem to mean that we

eat less at meal times; it just whets the appetite.

Eating throughout the day is now so normal, so much the expected thing to do, that it is almost shocking to suggest there is value in doing the absolute opposite. When I first started fasting I discovered some unexpected things about myself, my attitudes to food and about my beliefs.

- I discovered that I often eat when I don't need to. I do it because the food is there, because I am afraid that I will get hungry later, or simply from habit

- I assumed that when you get hungry it builds and builds until it becomes intolerable, and so you bury your face in a vat of ice cream. I found instead that hunger passes and once you have been really hungry you no longer fear it

- I thought that fasting would make me distractible, unable to concentrate. What I've discovered is that it sharpens my senses and my brain

- I wondered if I would feel faint for much of the time. It turns out that the body is incredibly adaptable and many athletes I've spoken to advocate training while fasting

- I feared it would be incredibly hard to do. It isn't

Why I got started

Although most of the great religions advocate fasting (the Sikhs are an exception, though they do allow fasting for medical reasons), I have always assumed that this was principally a way of testing yourself and your faith. I could see potential spiritual benefits but I was deeply sceptical about the physical benefits.

I have also had a number of body-conscious friends who, down the years, have tried to get me to fast, but I could never accept their explanation that the reason for doing so was 'to rest the liver' or 'to remove the toxins'. Neither explanation made any sense to a medically trained sceptic like me. I remember one friend telling me that after a couple of weeks of fasting his urine had turned black, proof that the toxins were leaving. I saw it as proof that he was an ignorant hippy and that whatever was going on inside his body as a result of fasting was extremely damaging. As I wrote in the introduction, what convinced me to try fasting was a combination of my own personal circumstances – in my mid-50s, high blood sugar, slightly overweight – and the emerging scientific evidence, which I list below.

That which does not kill us makes us stronger

There were a number of researchers who inspired me in

their different ways, but one who stands out is Professor Mark Mattson of the National Institute on Aging in Baltimore. A couple of years ago he wrote an article with Edward Calabrese in *New Scientist* magazine, 'When a little poison is good for you',[2] which really made me sit up and think.

'A little poison is good for you' is a colourful way of describing the theory of hormesis – the idea that when a human, or indeed any other creature, is exposed to a stress or toxin it can toughen them up. Hormesis is not just a variant of 'join the army and it will make a man of you'; it is now a well-accepted explanation in biology of how things operate at the cellular level.

Take, for example, something as simple as exercise. When you run or pump iron, what you are actually doing is damaging your muscles, causing small tears and rips. If you don't completely overdo it, then your body responds by doing repairs and in the process makes the muscles stronger.

Vegetables are another example. We all know that we should eat lots of fruit and vegetables because they are chock full of antioxidants – and antioxidants are great because they mop up the dangerous free radicals that roam our bodies doing harm.

The trouble with this widely accepted explanation of how fruit and vegetables 'work' is that it is almost certainly wrong, or at least incomplete. The levels of antioxidants in fruits and vegetables are far too low to have the profound effects they clearly do. In addition, the attempts to extract antioxidants from plants and then give them to us in a concentrated form, as a health-inducing supplement, have been unconvincing when tested in long-term trials. Betacarotene, when you get it in the form of a carrot, is undoubtedly good for you. When they took betacarotene out of the carrot and gave it as a supplement to patients with cancer, it actually seemed to make them worse.

If we look through the prism of hormesis at the way vegetables work in our bodies, we can see that the reasons for their benefits may be quite different.

Consider this apparent paradox: bitterness is often associated in the wild with poisons, something to be avoided. Plants produce a huge range of so-called phytochemicals and some of them act as natural pesticides, to keep mammals like us from eating them. The fact that they taste bitter is a clear warning signal: keep away. So there are good evolutionary reasons why we should dislike and avoid bitter-tasting foods. Yet some of the vegetables that are particularly good for us, such as cabbage, cauliflower, broccoli and other members of the brassica family, are so bitter that even as adults many of us struggle to love them.

The resolution to this paradox is that these vegetables taste bitter because they contain chemicals that are potentially poisonous. The reason they don't harm us is that these chemicals are present in them at low doses that are not toxic. Rather, they activate stress responses and switch on genes that protect and repair.

Once you start looking at the world in this way, you realise that many activities we initially find stressful – like eating bitter vegetables, going for a run, or Intermittent Fasting – are far from harmful. The challenge itself seems to be part of the benefit. The fact that prolonged starvation is clearly very bad for you does not imply that short periods of Intermittent Fasting must be a little bit bad for you. Indeed the reverse is true.

This point was vividly made to me by Professor Valter Longo, director of the University of Southern California's Longevity Institute. His research is mainly into the study of why we age, particularly concerning approaches that reduce the risk of developing age-related diseases such as cancer and diabetes.

I went to see Valter, not just because he is a world expert, but also because he had kindly agreed to act as my fasting mentor and buddy, to help inspire and guide me through my first experience of fasting.

Valter has been studying fasting for many years, and he is a keen adherent of it. He lives by his research and thrives on the sort of low-protein, high-vegetable diet that his grandparents enjoy in southern Italy. Perhaps not coincidentally, his grandparents live in a part of Italy that has an extraordinarily high concentration of long-lived people.

As well as following a fairly strict diet, Valter skips

lunch to keep his weight down. Beyond this, once every six months or so, he does a prolonged fast that lasts several days. Tall, slim, energetic, Italian, he is an inspiring poster boy for would-be fasters.

The main reason he is so enthusiastic about fasting is that his research, and that of others, has demonstrated the extraordinary range of measurable health benefits that you get from doing it. Going without food for even quite short periods of time switches on a number of 'repair genes', which, as he explained, can confer long-term benefits. 'There is a lot of initial evidence to suggest that temporary periodic fasting can induce long-lasting changes that can be beneficial against ageing and diseases,' he told me. 'You take a person, you fast them, after 24 hours everything is revolutionised. And even if you took a cocktail of drugs, very potent drugs, you will never even get close to what fasting does. The beauty of fasting is that it's all co-ordinated.'

Fasting and longevity

Most of the early long-term studies on the benefits of fasting were done in rodents. They also gave us important insights into the molecular mechanisms that underpin fasting.

In one early study from 1945, mice were fasted for either one day in four, one day in three or one day in two.

The researchers found that the fasted mice lived longer than a control group, and that the more they fasted the longer they lived. They also found that, unlike calorie-restricted mice, the fasted mice were not physically stunted.[3]

Since then numerous studies have confirmed, at least in rodents, the value of fasting. But why does fasting help? What is the mechanism?

Valter has access to his own supply of genetically engineered mice, known as dwarf or Laron mice, which he was keen to show me. These mice, though small, hold the record for longevity extension in a mammal. In other words, they live for an astonishingly long time.

The average mouse doesn't live that long, perhaps two years. Laron mice can live twice that, many for over four years when they are also calorie-restricted. In a human, that would be the equivalent of reaching almost 170.

The fascinating thing about Laron mice is not just their longevity, but the fact that they stay healthy for most of their very long lives. They simply don't seem to be prone to diabetes or cancer, and when they die, more often than not, it is of natural causes. Valter told me that on autopsy they are often unable to find a cause of death. They just seem to drop dead.

The reason these mice are so small and so long-lived is that they are genetically engineered so that their bodies do not respond to a hormone called IGF-1, Insulin-Like Growth Factor 1. IGF-1, as its name implies, has growth-promoting effects on almost every cell in your body. It keeps your cells constantly active. You need adequate levels of IGF-1 and other growth factors when you are young and growing, but high levels later in life appear to lead to accelerated ageing and cancer. As Valter put it, it's like driving along with your foot flat down on the accelerator, pushing the car to continue to perform all the time. 'Imagine, instead of occasionally taking your car to the garage and changing parts and pieces, you simply kept on driving it and driving it and driving it. Well, the car, of course, is going to break down.'

Valter's work is focused on trying to figure out how you can go on driving as much as possible, and as fast as possible, while enjoying life. He thinks the answer is periodic fasting. Because one of the ways fasting works is by making your body reduce the amount of IGF-1 it produces.

The evidence that IGF-1 plays a key role in many of the diseases of ageing comes not just from rodents like the Laron mice but also from humans. For the last seven years, Valter has been studying villagers in Ecuador with a genetic defect, also called Laron syndrome. This is an extremely rare condition which affects fewer than 350 people in the world. People with Laron syndrome have bodies which don't seem to be able to respond to IGF-1. There's a specific mutation in the growth hormone receptor, causing a deficiency that is very similar to that in the Laron mouse.

The villagers with Laron syndrome are normally quite short; many are less than four feet tall. The thing that is most surprising about them, however, is that, like the Laron mice, they simply don't seem to develop common diseases like diabetes and cancer. In fact, Valter says that, though they have been studied for many years, there is not a single case he has come across of someone with Laron dying of cancer. Yet their relatives, who live in the same household but who don't have Laron syndrome, get cancer like everybody else.

Disappointingly, for anyone hoping that IGF-1 will provide the secrets of immortality, people with Laron syndrome, unlike the mice, are not exceptionally long-lived. They certainly lead long lives, but not super-long lives. Valter thinks one reason for this may be that they tend to enjoy life rather than worry about their lifestyle. 'They smoke, eat a high-calorie diet, and then they look at me and they say, "Oh it doesn't matter, I'm immune."'

Valter thinks they prefer the idea of living as they want and dying at 85, rather than living more carefully and perhaps going beyond 100. He would like to persuade some of them to take on a healthy lifestyle and see what happens, but knows he wouldn't live long enough to see the outcome.

Fasting and repair genes

As well as reducing circulating levels of IGF-1, fasting also appears to switch on a number of repair genes. The reason this happens is not fully understood, but the evolutionary argument goes something like this. As long as we have plenty of food, our bodies are mainly interested in growing, having sex and reproducing. Nature has no long-term plans for us. She does not invest in our old age. Once we have reproduced we become disposable.

So what happens if you decide to fast? Well, the body's initial reaction is one of shock. Signals go to the brain reminding you that you are hungry, urging you to go out and find something to eat. But you resist. The body now decides that the reason you are not eating as much and as frequently as you usually do must be because you are now in a famine situation. In the past this would have been quite normal.

In a famine situation there is no point in expending energy on growth or sex. Instead the wisest thing the body can do is spend its precious store of energy on repair, trying to keep you in reasonable shape until the good times return once more. The result is that, as well as removing its foot from the accelerator, your body takes itself along to the cellular equivalent of a garage. There, all the little gene mechanics are ordered to start doing some of the urgent maintenance tasks that have been put off till now.

One of the things that calorie restriction does, for example, is to switch on a process called autophagy.[4] Autophagy, meaning 'self eat', is a process by which the body breaks down and recycles old and tired cells; just as with a car, it is important to get rid of damaged or ageing parts if you are going to keep things in good working order.

Valter thinks that the majority of people with a BMI over 25 would benefit from fasting, but he also thinks that if you plan to do it for more than a day it should be done in a proper centre. As he put it, 'a prolonged fast is an extreme intervention. If it's done well, it can be very powerful in your favour. If it's done improperly, it can be very powerful against you.' With a prolonged fast lasting several days, you also get a drop in blood pressure and some fairly profound metabolic re-programming. Some people faint. It's not common but it happens.

One of Valter's areas of research is into the effects of fasting on cancer (see more on pages 56-7 below) and this seems to be optimised by prolonged rather than Intermittent Fasting . As he pointed out, the first time you try fasting for a few days it can be a bit of a struggle. 'Our bodies are used to high levels of glucose and high levels of insulin, so it takes time to adapt. But then eventually it's not that hard.'

I wasn't keen to hear 'eventually', but by then I knew I would have to give it a go. It was a challenge, and one I thought I could win. Brain against stomach. No contest.

Experiencing a four-day fast

I don't think it is either necessary or particularly desirable to do a prolonged fast before embarking on the Fast Diet. While there are few known risks involved in fasting for less than 24 hours, the same is not true of prolonged fasts. I decided to start with a four-day fast because I knew I was in safe hands. I had also had my IGF-1 levels measured just before I met Valter and they were high. Not super-high, as he kindly put it, but at the top end of the range (my levels of IGF-1 or somatomedin-C, as it's also known, were 28.0nmol/l. The healthy range is 11.3–30.9nmol/l).

High levels of IGF-1 are associated with a range of cancers, among them prostate cancer which had troubled my father. Would a four-day fast change anything?

I had been warned that the first few days might be tough, but after that I would start feeling the effects of a rush of what Valter termed 'wellbeing chemicals'. Even better, the next time I fasted it would be easier because my body and brain would have a memory of it and understand what I was going through.

Having decided that I would try an extended fast, my next decision was how harsh to make it. A number of different countries have a tradition of fasting. The Russians seem to prefer it tough. For them, a fast consists of nothing but water, cold showers and exercise. The Germans, on the other hand, prefer their fasts to be considerably gentler. Go to a fasting clinic in Germany and you will probably be fed around 200 calories a day in comfortable surroundings.

I wanted to see results, so I went for a British compromise. I would eat 25 calories a day, no cold showers and just try working as normal.

So on a warm Monday evening, I enjoyed my last meal, a filling dinner of steak, chips and salad washed down with beer. I felt a certain trepidation as I realised that for the next four days I would be drinking nothing but water, sugarless black tea and coffee, and one measly cup of low-calorie soup a day.

Despite what I'd been told and read, before I began my fast I secretly feared that hunger would grow and grow, gnawing away inside me until I finally gave in and ran amok in a cakeshop. The first 24 hours were quite tough, just as Valter had predicted, but as he had also predicted things got better, not worse. Yes, there were hunger pangs, sometimes quite distracting, but if I kept busy they went away.

During the first 24 hours of a fast, there are some quite profound changes going on inside the body. Within a few hours, glucose circulating in the blood is consumed. If that's not being replaced by food then the body turns to glycogen, a stable form of glucose that is stored in the muscles and liver.

Only when that's gone does it really switch on fat burning. What actually happens is that fatty acids are broken down in the liver, resulting in the production of something called ketone bodies. The brain uses these ketone bodies as a source of energy, instead of glucose.

The first two days of a fast can be uncomfortable because your body and brain are having to cope with the switch from using glucose and glycogen as a fuel to using ketone bodies. The body is not used to them so you can get headaches, though I didn't. You may find it hard to sleep. I didn't. The biggest problem I had with fasting is hard to put into words; it was sometimes just feeling 'uncomfortable'. I can't really describe it more accurately than that. I didn't feel faint; I just felt out of place.

I did, occasionally, feel hungry, but most of the time I was surprisingly cheerful. By day three the feel-good hormones had come to my rescue.

By Friday, day four, I was almost disappointed that it was ending. Almost. Despite Valter's warning that it would be unwise to gorge immediately on breaking a fast, I got myself a plate of bacon and eggs and settled down to eat. After a few mouthfuls I was full. I really didn't need any more and in fact skipped lunch.

That afternoon I was tested again and discovered I had lost just under three pounds of body weight, a significant portion of which was fat. I was also happy to see that my blood glucose levels had fallen substantially and that my IGF-1 levels, which had been at the top end of the recommended range, had gone right down. In fact, they had almost halved. This was all good news.

I had lost some fat, my blood results were looking good, and I had learnt that I can control my hunger. Valter was extremely pleased with these changes, particularly the fall in IGF-1 that he said would significantly reduce my risk of cancer. But he also warned me that if I went back to my old lifestyle these changes would not be permanent.

Valter's research points towards the fact that high levels of protein, the amounts found in a typical western diet, help keep IGF-1 levels high. I knew that there is protein in foods like meat and fish, but I was surprised that there is so much in milk. I used to like drinking a skinny latte most mornings. I had the illusion that because it is made with skimmed milk it is healthy. Unfortunately, though low in fat, a large latte comes in at around 11g of protein. And Valter recommends that you don't eat more than 0.8g of protein per kg of body weight per day. For someone like me, that would be around 64g a day. The lattes would have to go.

Fasting and weight loss

One way to lose weight would be to go on a prolonged fast. I did the four-day fast, as described above, mainly because I was curious. I would not recommend it as a weight-loss regime because it is completely unsustainable. Unless they combine it with a vigorous exercise regime, people who go on prolonged fasts lose muscle as well as fat. Then, when they stop, as they must eventually do, the risk is they will pile the weight right back on.

Fortunately less drastic, Intermittent Fasting – the subject of this book – leads to steady and sustainable weight loss and does not cause muscle loss.

Alternate Day Fasting

One of the most extensively studied forms of short-term fasting is Alternate Day Fasting (ADF). As its name implies, it means you get no food, or relatively little food, every other day. One of the few researchers to have done human studies in this area is Dr Krista Varady of the University of Illinois at Chicago.

Krista is slim, charming and very amusing. We met in an old-fashioned American diner where I guiltily ate burgers and fries while Krista told me about one of the recent studies she has been carrying out with human volunteers.[5] On fasting days the volunteers were allowed 25% of their normal energy needs, so men were allowed around 600 calories a day, women 500 calories a day. On fast days they ate all their calories in one go, at lunch. On their feed days they were asked to consume 125% of their normal energy needs.

Krista has done a number of studies on ADF, and what surprised her is that, even when they are allowed to, people don't go crazy on their feed days. 'I thought when I started running these trials that people would eat 175% the next day; they'd just fully compensate and wouldn't lose any weight. But most people eat around 110%, just slightly over what they usually eat. I haven't measured it yet, but I think it involves stomach size, how far that can expand out. Because eating almost twice the amount of food that you normally eat is actually pretty difficult. You can do it over time; people that are obese, their stomachs get bigger to accommodate, you know, 5000 calories a day. But just to do it right off is actually pretty difficult.'

In her earlier studies, subjects were asked to stick to a low-fat diet, but what Krista wanted to know was whether ADF would also work if her subjects were allowed to eat a typical American high-fat diet. So she asked 33 obese volunteers, most of them women, to go on ADF for eight weeks. Before starting, the volunteers were divided into two groups. One group was put on a low-fat diet, eating low-fat cheeses and dairies, very lean meats and a lot of fruit and vegetables. The other group was allowed to eat high-fat lasagnes, pizza, the sort of diet a typical American might consume. Americans consume somewhere between 35 and 45% fat in their diet.

As Krista explained, the results were unexpected. The researchers and volunteers had assumed that the people on the low-fat diet would lose more weight than those on the high-fat diet. But, if anything, it was the other way around. The volunteers on the high-fat diet lost an average of 5.6kg, while those on the low-fat diet lost 4.2kg. They both lost about seven centimetres around their waists.

Krista thinks that the main reason this happened was compliance. The volunteers randomised to the high-fat diet were more likely to stick to it than those on the low-fat diet simply because they found it a lot more palatable. And it wasn't just weight loss. Both groups saw impressive falls in low-density lipoprotein (LDL) cholesterol, the bad cholesterol, and in blood pressure. This meant that they had reduced their risk of cardiovascular disease, of having a heart attack or stroke.

Krista doesn't want to encourage people to binge on rubbish. She would much rather that people on ADF ate healthily, increased their fruit and vegetable intake, and generally ate less. The trouble is, as she pointed out rather exasperatedly, doctors have been encouraging people to embrace a healthy lifestyle for decades, and not enough of us are doing it. She thinks dieticians should take into account what people actually do rather than what we would like them to do.

One other significant benefit to Intermittent Fasting is that you don't seem to lose muscle, which you would on a normal calorie-restricted regime. Krista herself is not sure why that is and wants to do further research.

The two-day fast

One of the problems with ADF, which is why I am not so keen on it, is that you have to do it every other day. In my experience this can be socially inconvenient as well as emotionally demanding. There is no pattern to your week and other people, friends and family, find it hard to keep track of when your fast and feed days are. Unlike Krista's subjects, I was not particularly overweight to start with, so I also worried about losing too much weight too rapidly. That is why, having tried ADF for a short while, I decided to cut back to fasting two days a week.

I now have my own experience of this to fall back on (see page 60), together with the experiences of hundreds of others who have written to me over the last few months. But what trials have been done on two-day fasts in humans?

Well, Dr Michelle Harvie, a dietician based at the Genesis Breast Cancer Prevention Centre at the Wythenshawe Hospital in Manchester, has done a number of studies assessing the effects of a two-day fast on female volunteers. In a recent study, she divided 115 women into three groups. One group was asked to stick to a 1500-calorie Mediterranean diet, and was also encouraged to avoid high-fat foods and alcohol.[6] Another group was asked to eat normally five days a week, but to eat a 650-calorie, low-carbohydrate diet on the other two days. A final group was asked to avoid carbohydrates for two days a week, but was otherwise not calorie-restricted.

After three months, the women on the two-day diets had lost an average of 4kg, which was almost twice as much as the full-time dieters, who had lost an average of just 2.4kg. Insulin resistance had also improved significantly in the two-day diet groups (see more on insulin on page 54).

The focus of Michelle's work is trying to reduce breast cancer risk through dietary interventions. Being obese and having high levels of insulin resistance are both risk factors. On the Genesis website (www.genesisuk.org), she points out that they have been studying Intermittent Fasting at the Genesis Breast Cancer Prevention Centre, University Hospital of South Manchester NHS Foundation Trust, for over six years and that their research has shown that cutting down on your calories for two days a week gives the same benefits, possibly more, than by going on a normal calorie-reduced diet. 'To date, our research has concluded that intermittent diets appear to be a safe, viable, alternative approach to weight loss and maintaining a lower weight, in comparison to daily dieting.'

Is it just calories?

If you eat 500 or 600 calories two days a week and don't significantly overcompensate during the rest of the week, then you will lose weight in a steady fashion.

But is there any evidence that Intermittent Fasting does more than that? I recently came across one particularly fascinating study suggesting that when you eat can be almost as important as what you eat.

In this study, scientists from the Salk Institute for Biological Studies took two groups of mice and fed them a high-fat diet.[7] The mice got exactly the same amount of food to eat, the only difference being that one group of mice was allowed to eat whenever they wanted, nibbling away when they were in the mood, rather like we do, while the other group of mice had to eat their food in an eight-hour time period. This meant that there were 16 hours of the day in which they were, involuntarily, fasting.

After 100 days, there were some truly dramatic differences between the two groups of mice. The mice who nibbled away at their fatty food had developed high cholesterol, high blood glucose and had liver damage. The mice that had been forced to fast for 16 hours a day put on far less weight (28% less) and suffered much less liver damage, despite having eaten exactly the same amount and quality of food. They also had lower levels of chronic inflammation, which suggests they had reduced risk of a number of diseases, including heart disease, cancer, stroke and Alzheimer's.

The Salk researchers' explanation for this is that all the time you are eating your insulin levels are elevated and your body is stuck in fat-storing mode (see the discussion of insulin on page 54). Only after a few hours of fasting is your body able to turn off the 'fat storing' and turn on the 'fat burning' mechanisms. So if you are a mouse and you are continually nibbling, your body will just continue making and storing fat, resulting in obesity and liver damage.

By now, I hope you are as convinced as I am that fasting offers multiple health benefits, as well as helping to achieve weight loss. I had been aware of some of these claims before I got really interested in fasting and, though initially sceptical, I was converted by the sheer weight of evidence.

But there was one area of study that was a complete surprise: research showing how fasting can improve mood and protect the brain from dementia and cognitive decline. This, for me, was something completely new, unexpected, and hugely exciting.

Fasting and the brain

The brain, as Woody Allen once said, is my second favourite organ. I might even put it first, as without it nothing else would function. The human brain, around three pounds of pinkish greyish gunk with the consistency of tapioca, has been described as the most complex object in the known universe. It allows us to build, write poetry, dominate the planet and even understand ourselves, something no other creature has succeeded in doing.

It is also an extremely efficient energy-saving machine, doing all that complicated thinking and making sure our bodies are functioning properly while using the same amount of energy as a 25-watt light bulb. The fact that our brains are normally so flexible and adaptable makes it even more tragic when they go wrong. I am aware that as I get older my memory has become more fallible. I've compensated by using a range of memory tricks I've picked up over the years, but even so I find myself occasionally struggling to remember names and dates. Far worse than this, however, is the fear that one day I may lose my mind entirely, perhaps developing some form of dementia. Obviously I want to preserve my brain in as good a shape as possible and for as long as possible. Fortunately fasting seems to offer significant protection.

The man I went to discuss my brain with was Professor Mark Mattson.

Mark Mattson, a professor of neuroscience at the National Institute on Aging, is one of the most revered scientists in his field: the study of the ageing brain. I find his work genuinely inspiring – suggesting, as it does, that fasting can help combat diseases like Alzheimer's, dementia and memory loss.

Although I could have taken a taxi to his office, I chose to walk. I'm a fan of walking. It not only burns calories, it also improves the mood, and it may also help retain your memory. Normally as we get older our brain shrinks, but one study found that in regular walkers the hippocampus, an area of the brain essential for memory, actually expanded.[8] Regular walkers have brains that in MRI scans look, on average, two years younger than the brains of those who are sedentary.

Mark, who studies Alzheimer's, lost his own father to dementia. He told me that although it didn't directly motivate him to go into this particular line of research – when he started work on Alzheimer's disease his father had not yet been diagnosed – but it did give him insight.

Alzheimer's affects around 26 million people worldwide and the problem will grow as the population ages. New approaches are desperately needed because the tragedy of Alzheimer's disease and other forms of dementia is that once you're diagnosed it may be possible to delay, but not prevent, the inevitable deterioration. You are likely to get progressively worse to the point where you need constant care for many years. By the end you may not even recognise the faces of those you once loved.

Can fasting make you clever?

Just as Valter Longo had, Mark took me off to see some mice. Like Valter's mice, Mark's mice are genetically engineered, But they have been modified to make them more vulnerable to Alzheimer's. The mice I saw were in a maze, which they had to navigate in order to find food. Some of the mice perform this task with relative ease; others get disorientated and confused. This task, and others like it, are designed to reveal signs that the mice are developing memory problems; a mouse that is struggling will quickly forget which arm of the maze it has already travelled down.

The genetically engineered Alzheimer's mice will, if put on a normal diet, quickly develop dementia. By the time they are a year old, the equivalent of middle age in humans, they normally have obvious learning and memory problems. The animals put on an intermittent fast, something Mark prefers to call 'intermittent energy restriction', often go up to 20 months without any detectable signs of dementia.[9] They only really start deteriorating towards the end of their lives. In humans that would be the equivalent of developing signs of Alzheimer's at the age of 80 rather than at 50. I know which I would prefer.

Disturbingly, when these mice are put on a typical junk-food diet, they go downhill much earlier than even normally fed mice. 'We put mice on a high-fat and high-fructose diet,' Mark said, 'and that has a dramatic effect; the animals have an earlier onset of the learning and memory problems, more accumulation of amyloid and more problems with finding their way in a maze test.'

In other words, junk food makes these mice fat and stupid.

One of the key changes that occur in the brains of

Mark's fasting mice is increased production of a protein called brain-derived neurotrophic factor. BDNF has been shown to stimulate stem cells to turn into new nerve cells in the hippocampus. As I mentioned earlier, this is a part of the brain that is essential for normal learning and memory.

But why should the hippocampus grow in response to fasting? Mark points out that from an evolutionary perspective it makes sense. After all, the times when you need to be smart and on the ball are when there's not a lot of food lying around. 'If an animal is in an area where there's limited food resources, it's important that they are able to remember where food is, remember where hazards are, predators and so on. We think that people in the past who were able to respond to hunger with increased cognitive ability had a survival advantage.'

We don't know for sure if humans grow new brain cells in response to fasting; to be absolutely certain researchers would need to put volunteers on an intermittent fast and then kill them, take their brains out and look for signs of new neural growth. It seems unlikely that many would volunteer for such a project. But what they are doing is a study where volunteers fast and then MRI scans are used to see if the size of their hippocampi changes over time.

As I mentioned above, these techniques have been used in humans to show that regular exercise, such as walking, increases the size of the hippocampus. Hopefully similar studies will show that two days a week of Intermittent Fasting is good for learning and memory. On a purely anecdotal level, and using a sample size of one, it seems to work. Before starting the Fast Diet, I did a sophisticated memory test online. Two months in I repeated the test and my performance had, indeed, improved. If you are interested in doing something similar then I suggest you go to www.cognitivefun.net/test/2. Do let us know how you get on.

Fasting and mood

One of the things that Professor Valter Longo and others told me before I began my four-day fast was that it would be tough initially, but that after a while I would start to feel more cheerful, which was indeed what happened. Similarly, I was surprised to discover how positive I have felt while doing Intermittent Fasting. I expected to feel tired and crabby on my fasting days, but not at all. So is this simply a psychological effect, that people who do Intermittent Fasting and lose weight feel good about themselves, or are there also chemical changes that are influencing mood?

According to Professor Mark Mattson, one of the reasons people may find Intermittent Fasting relatively easy to do due to its effects on BDNF. BDNF not only seems to protect the brain against the ravages of dementia and age-related mental decline, but it may also improve your mood.

There have been a number of studies going back many years that suggest rising levels of BDNF have an antidepressant effect, at least in rodents. In one study, they injected BDNF directly into the brains of rats and found this had similar effects to repeated use of a standard antidepressant.[10] Another paper found that electric shock therapy, which is known to be effective in severe depression, seems to work, at least in part, because it stimulates the production of higher levels of BDNF.[11]

Mark Mattson believes that within a few weeks of starting a two-day-a-week fasting regime, BDNF levels will start to rise, suppressing anxiety and elevating mood. He doesn't currently have the human data to fully support this claim, but he is doing trials on volunteers which involve, among other things, collecting regular samples of cerebrospinal fluid (the liquid that bathes the brain) in order to measure the changes that occur during intermittent fasts. This is not a trial for the faint-hearted as it requires regular spinal taps, but as Mark pointed out to me, many of his volunteers are already undergoing early signs of cognitive change, so they are extremely motivated.

Mark is keen to study and promote the benefits of Intermittent Fasting as he is genuinely worried about the likely effects of the current obesity epidemic on our brains and our society. He also thinks if that if you are considering Intermittent Fasting you should get going sooner rather than later: 'The age-related cognitive decline in Alzheimer's disease, the events that are occurring in the brain at the level of the nerve cells and the molecules in the nerve cells, those changes are occurring very early, probably decades before the subject starts to have learning and memory problems. That's why it's critical to start dietary regimes early on, when people are young or middle-aged, so that they can slow down the development of these processes in the brain and live to be 90 with their brain functioning perfectly well.'

Like Mark, I'm convinced the human brain benefits from short periods abstaining from food. This is an exciting and fast-emerging area of research that many will watch with great interest. Beyond the brain, though, Intermittent Fasting also has measurable, beneficial effects on other areas of the body – on your heart, on your blood profile, on your risk of cancer. And that's where we'll turn now.

Fasting and the heart

One of the main reasons I decided to try fasting was that tests had suggested I was heading for serious problems with my cardiovascular system. Nothing has happened yet, but the warning signs were flashing amber. The tests showed that my blood levels of LDL (low-density lipoprotein, the 'bad' cholesterol) were disturbingly high, as were the levels of my fasting glucose.

To measure 'fasting glucose' you have to fast overnight, then give a sample of blood. The normal, desirable range is 3.9-5.8mmol/l. Mine was 7.3mmol/l. Not yet diabetic, but dangerously high. There are many reasons why you should do all you can to avoid becoming a diabetic, not least the fact that it dramatically increases your risk of having a heart attack or stroke.

Fasting glucose is an important thing to measure because it is an indicator that all may not be well with your insulin levels.

Insulin – the fat-making hormone

When we eat food, particularly food rich in carbohydrates, our blood glucose levels rise and the pancreas, an organ below the ribs and near the left kidney, starts to churn out insulin. Glucose is the main fuel that our cells use for energy, but the body does not like having high levels of it circulating in the blood. The job of insulin, a hormone, is to regulate blood glucose levels, ensuring that they are neither too high nor too low. It normally does this with great precision. The problem comes when the pancreas gets overloaded.

Insulin is a sugar controller; it aids the extraction of

glucose from blood and then stores it in places like your liver or muscles in a stable form called glycogen, to be used when and if it is needed. What is less commonly known is that insulin is also a fat controller. It inhibits something called lipolysis, the release of stored body fat. At the same time, it forces fat cells to take up and store fat from your blood. Insulin makes you fat. High levels lead to increased fat storage, low levels to fat depletion.

The trouble with constantly eating lots of sugary, carbohydrate-rich foods and drinks, as we increasingly do, is that this requires the release of more and more insulin to deal with the glucose surge. Up to a point, your pancreas will cope by simply pumping out ever-larger quantities of insulin. This leads to greater fat deposition and also increases the risk of cancer. Naturally enough, this can't go on forever. If you continue to produce ever-larger quantities of insulin, your cells will eventually rebel and become resistant to its effects. It's rather like shouting at your children; you can keep escalating things, but after a certain point they will simply stop listening.

Eventually the cells stop responding to insulin; your blood glucose levels now stay permanently high and you will find you have joined the 285 million people around the world who have type 2 diabetes. It is a massive and rapidly growing problem worldwide. Over the last 20 years, numbers have risen almost tenfold and there is no obvious sign that this trend is slowing.

Diabetes is associated with an increased risk of heart attack, stroke, impotence, going blind and losing your extremities due to poor circulation. It is also associated with brain shrinkage and dementia. Not a pretty picture.

One way to prevent the downward spiral into diabetes is to cut back on the carbohydrates and instead start eating more vegetables and fat, since these foods do not lead to such big spikes in blood glucose. Nor do they have such a dramatic effect on insulin levels. The other way is to try Intermittent Fasting.

How Intermittent Fasting affects insulin sensitivity

In a study from 2005, eight healthy young men were asked to fast every other day, 20 hours a day, for two weeks.[12] On their fasting days they were allowed to eat until 10pm, then not eat again until 6pm the following evening. They were also asked to eat heartily the rest of the time to make sure they did not lose any weight.

The idea behind the experiment was to test the so-called 'thrifty hypothesis', the idea that since we evolved at a time of feast and famine the best way to eat is to mimic those times. At the end of the two weeks, there were no changes in the volunteers' weight or body-fat composition, which is what the researchers had intended. There was, however, a big change in their insulin sensitivity. In other words, after just two weeks of Intermittent Fasting, the same amount of circulating insulin now had a much greater effect on the volunteers' ability to store glucose or break down fat.

The researchers wrote jubilantly that, 'by subjecting healthy men to cycles of feast and famine we changed their metabolic status for the better'. They also added that, 'to our knowledge this is the first study in humans in which an increased insulin action on whole body glucose uptake and adipose tissue lipolysis has been obtained by means of Intermittent Fasting.'

I don't know what impact Intermittent Fasting has had on my insulin sensitivity – it's a test that is hard to do and extremely expensive – but what I do know is that the effects on my blood sugar have been spectacular. Before I started fasting, my blood glucose level was 7.3 mmol/l, well above the acceptable range of 3.9 – 5.8 mmol/l. The last time I had my level measured it was 5.0 mmol/l, still a bit high but well within the normal range.

This is an incredibly impressive response. My doctor, who was preparing to put me on medication, was astonished at such a dramatic turnaround. Doctors routinely recommend a healthy diet to patients with high blood glucose, but it usually only makes a marginal difference. Intermittent Fasting could have a revolutionary, game-changing effect on the nation's health.

Fasting and cancer

My father was a lovely man but not a particularly healthy one. Overweight for much of his life, by the time he reached his 60s he had developed not only diabetes but also prostate cancer. He had an operation to remove the cancer that left him with embarrassing urinary problems. Understandably, I am not at all keen to go down that road.

My four-day fast, under Professor Valter Longo's supervision, had shown me that it was possible to dramatically cut my IGF-1 (Insulin-like Growth Factor 1) levels and by doing so, hopefully, my prostate cancer risk. I later discovered that Intermittent Fasting had a similar effect on my IGF-1 levels. The link between growth, fasting and cancer is worth unpacking.

The cells in our bodies are constantly multiplying, replacing dead, worn-out or damaged tissue. This is fine as long as cellular growth is under control, but sometimes a cell mutates, grows uncontrollably and turns into a cancer. Very high levels in the blood of a cellular stimulant, like IGF-1, are likely to increase the chance of this happening.

When a cancer goes rogue, the normal options are surgery, chemotherapy or radiotherapy. Surgery is used to try to remove the tumour; chemotherapy and radiotherapy are there to try and poison it. The major problem with chemotherapy and radiotherapy is that they are not selective; as well as killing tumour cells they will kill or damage surrounding healthy cells. They are particularly likely to damage rapidly dividing cells such as hair roots, which is why hair commonly falls out following therapy.

As I mentioned above, Valter Longo has shown that when we are deprived of food for even quite short periods of time, our body responds by slowing things down, going into repair and survival mode until food is once more abundant. That is true of normal cells. But cancer cells follow their own rules. They are, almost by definition, not under control and will go on selfishly proliferating whatever the circumstances. This 'selfishness' creates an opportunity. If you fast just before chemotherapy, at least in theory, you create a situation where your normal cells are hibernating while the cancer cells are running amok and therefore more vulnerable.

In a paper published in 2008, Valter and colleagues showed that fasting 'protects normal but not cancer cells against high-dose chemotherapy'.[13] They followed this with another paper in which they showed that fasting increased the efficacy of chemotherapy drugs against a variety of cancers.[14]

Again, as is so often the case, this was a study done with mice. But the implications of Valter's work were not missed by an eagle-eyed judge called Nora Quinn, who saw a short article about it in *The LA Times*.

Nora's story

I met Nora in Los Angeles. She is a feisty woman with a terrific, dry sense of humour. Nora first noticed she had a problem when, one morning, she put her hand on her breast and felt a lump the size of a walnut under her skin. After indulging, as she put it, in the fantasy that it was a cyst, it was removed and sent to a pathologist.

'The reality of your life always comes out in pathology,' she told me. When the pathology report came back it said that she had invasive breast cancer. She had a course of radiotherapy and was about to start chemotherapy when she read about Professor Longo's work with mice.

She tried to speak to Valter, but he wouldn't advise her because none of the trials he had run, up to that point, had been done with humans. He didn't know if it was safe for someone about to undergo chemo to fast and he certainly wasn't going to encourage people like Nora to give it a go.

Undeterred, Nora did her own research and decided to try fasting for a seven-and-a-half-day, water-only fast; it would cover before, during and after chemotherapy. Having discovered how tough it can be to do even a four-day fast while fully healthy, I'm surprised she was able to go through with it, though Nora says it's not so hard and I'm just a wimp. The results were mixed: 'After the first chemo I didn't get that sick, but my hair fell out.'

So next time she didn't fast, and she was only medium

sick. 'I thought it wasn't working. I thought, seven and a half days of fasting to avoid being medium sick, this is a really bad deal. I am so not doing that again.'

When it was time for her third course of chemo, she didn't fast. That, she now feels, was a mistake.

'I got sick. I don't have words for how sick I was. I was weak, felt poisoned, and I couldn't get up. I felt like I was moving through jello. It was absolutely horrible.'

The cells that line the gut, like hair root cells, grow rapidly because they need to be constantly replaced. That's one reason why chemotherapy can make people feel really ill.

By the time Nora had to undergo her fourth course of chemo she had decided once again to try fasting. This time things went much better and she made a good recovery. She is currently cancer free.

Nora is convinced she benefitted from fasting but it's hard to be sure because she wasn't part of a proper medical trial. Valter and colleagues at University of Southern California did, however, study what happened to her and 10 other patients with cancers who had also decided to put themselves on a fast.[15] All of them reported fewer and less severe symptoms after chemotherapy and most of them, including Nora, saw improvements in their blood results. The white cells and platelets, for example, recovered more rapidly when they had chemo in a fasted state than when they did not. But why did Nora go rogue? Why didn't she fast under proper supervision?

'I decided to fast based on years of information from animal testing. I do agree that if you are going to do crazy things like I do you should have medical supervision. But how? None of my doctors would listen to me.'

Nora's self-experiment could have gone wrong, which is just one reason why such maverick behaviour is not recommended. Her experience, however, and that of the other nine cancer patients, helped inspire further studies.

For example, Professor Valter Longo and his colleagues have recently completed Phase I of a clinical trial to see if fasting around the time of chemotherapy is safe, which it seems to be. The next thing is to assess whether it makes a measurable difference. At least ten other hospitals around the world are either doing or have agreed to do clinical trials. Go to our website for the latest updates.

Intermittent Fasting: my personal journey

As you've read, I started out by trying the four-day fast under Professor Valter Longo's supervision. But despite the improvements in my blood biochemistry and his obvious enthusiasm, I could not imagine doing lengthy fasts on a regular basis for the rest of my life. So what next? Well, having met Dr Krista Varady and learnt all about ADF (Alternate Day Fasting) I decided to give that a go.

After a short while, however, I realised that it was

just too tough, physically, socially and psychologically. I need some pattern in my life and not being able to tell without a calendar and lengthy calculations whether I could meet friends for dinner on a particular night was irksome. I also found fasting every other day just a little too challenging. I realise that many of Krista's volunteers do manage to stick to it, but they are in a trial situation and highly motivated. It is undoubtedly an effective way to lose weight rapidly and to get powerful changes to your biochemistry, but it was not for me. So I decided to try eating 600 calories for two days a week. It seemed a reasonable compromise and, more importantly, doable.

I tried eating all my food in one meal, but I discovered that if I skipped breakfast I started to feel hungry and irritable well before lunch. So I split my food in two: a moderate breakfast, miss lunch, a light supper. And I did it twice a week. This I found extremely manageable.

After experimenting with different versions of fasting, I found the 5:2 approach is the most effective and workable way for me to get the benefits of fasting and still retain a long-term commitment to a dietary plan. The 5:2 Fast Diet is based on a number of different forms of Intermittent Fasting; it is not based on any one body of research, but is a synthesis.

Before embarking on the diet, I decided to get myself properly tested, to see what effects it would have on my body. The following are the tests I did. Most are straightforward. The blood tests are, with one exception, tests your doctor should be happy to do for you.

Get on the scales

The first and most obvious thing you will want to do is weigh yourself before embarking on this adventure. Initially, it is best to do this at the same time every day. First thing in the morning is, as I'm sure you know, when you will be at your lightest.

Ideally you should get a weighing machine that measures body-fat percentage as well as weight, since what you really want to see is body-fat levels fall. The cheaper machines are not fantastically reliable; they tend to underestimate the true figure, giving you a false sense of security. What they are quite good at doing, however, is measuring change. In other words, they might tell you when you start that you are 30% body fat when the true figure is closer to 33%. But they should be able to tell you when that number begins to fall.

Body fat

Body fat is measured as a percentage of total weight. The machines you can buy do this by a system called impedence. There's a small electric current that runs through your body and the machine measures the resistance. It does its estimation based on the fact that muscle and other tissues are better conductors of electricity than fat.

The only way to get a truly accurate figure is with a machine called a DXA (formerly DEXA) scan. It stands for 'Dual Energy X-ray Absorptiometry'. It is expensive and for most people unnecessary. Your BMI will tell you if you are overweight. Women tend to have more body fat than men. A man with body fat of more than 25% would be considered overweight. For a woman it would be 30%.

Calculate your BMI
To calculate your BMI, go to a website such as www.nhs.uk/tools/pages/healthyweightcalculator.aspx. This will not only do the calculation, but also tell you what it means. One criticism of BMI is that someone who has a lot of muscle could get a high BMI score. This is not an issue for most of us. Sadly.

Measure your stomach
BMI is useful but it may not be the best predictor of future health. In a study of over 45,000 women followed for 16 years, the waist-to-height ratio was a superior predictor of who would develop heart disease. The reason why the waist matters so much is that visceral fat, which collects inside the abdomen, is the worst sort of fat, because it causes inflammation and puts you at much higher risk of diabetes. You don't need fancy equipment to tell you if you have internal fat. All you need is a tape measure.

Male or female, your waist should be less than half

your height. Most people underestimate their waist size by about two inches because they rely on trouser size. Instead, measure your waist by putting the tape measure around your belly button. Be honest. A definition of optimism is someone who steps on the scale, while holding their breath. You are fooling no one.

Blood tests

You should be able to get standard tests on the NHS.

> <u>Fasting glucose.</u> I chose to measure my fasting glucose because it is a really important measure of fitness, even if you are not at risk of diabetes, and a predictor of future health. Studies show that even moderately elevated levels of blood glucose are associated with increased risk of heart disease, stroke and long-term cognitive problems. Ideally I would have had my insulin sensitivity measured, but that test is complex and expensive.

> <u>Cholesterol.</u> They measure two types of cholesterol: LDL (low-density lipoprotein) and HDL (high-density lipoprotein). Broadly speaking, LDL carries cholesterol into the wall of your arteries while HDL

carries it away. It is good to have a low-ish LDL and a highish HDL. One way you can express this is as a percentage: HDL to HDL + LDL. Anything over 20% is good.

Triglycerides. These are a type of fat that is found in blood; they are one of the ways that the body stores calories. High levels are associated with increased risk of heart disease.

IGF-1. This is an expensive test and not available on the NHS. It is a measure of cell turnover and therefore of cancer risk. It may also be a marker for biological ageing. I wanted to find out the effects of 5:2 fasting on my IGF-1. I had discovered that IGF-1 levels drop dramatically in response to a four-day fast, but after a month of normal eating they bounced right back to where they had been before.

My data

These are the results of the physical measurements I took before starting the Fast Diet:

	ME	RECOMMENDED
HEIGHT	5' 11"	
WEIGHT	187lb	
BODY MASS INDEX	26.4	19-25
BODY FAT	28%	Less than 25% for men
WAIST SIZE	36 "	Less than half your height
NECK SIZE	17 "	Less than 16.5"

I wasn't obese, but both my BMI and my body-fat percentage told me that I was overweight. I knew from doing an MRI scan that much of my fat was collected internally, wrapping itself in thick layers around my liver and kidneys, disturbing all sorts of metabolic pathways.

Clearly, the fat wasn't all inside my abdomen. Quite a bit had collected around my neck. This meant that I was snoring. Loudly. Neck size is a powerful predictor of whether you will snore or not.[16] A neck size above 16.5" for men or 16 inches for women means you are in the danger zone.

	MY RESULTS in mmol/l	RECOMMENDED
DIABETES RISK: FASTING GLUCOSE	7.3	3.9–5.8
HEART DISEASE FACTORS: TRIGLYCERIDES HDL CHOLESTEROL LDL CHOLESTEROL	1.4 1.8 5.5	Less than 2.3 0.9–1.5 Up to 3.0

HEART DISEASE RISK HDL % of total	23%	20% and over
CANCER RISK Somatomedin-C (IGF-1)	28.6 nmol/l	11.3–30.9nmol/l

According to this data, my fasting glucose was worryingly high. I was not yet a diabetic but I had signs of what is called impaired glucose tolerance, pre-diabetes. My LDL was far too high, but I was to some extent protected by the fact that my triglycerides were low and my HDL high. This is not a good picture, though.

My IGF-1 levels were also too high, suggesting rapid turnover of cells and increased cancer risk.

After three months on the Fast Diet there were some remarkable changes.

	ME	RECOMMENDED
HEIGHT	5' 11"	
WEIGHT	168lb	
BODY MASS INDEX	24	19-25
BODY FAT	21%	Less than 25% for men
WAIST SIZE	33 inches	Less than half your height
NECK SIZE	16 inches	Less than 16.5 inches

I had lost about 19lb, almost one and a half stone. My BMI and body-fat percentage were now respectable. I had to go out and buy smaller belts and tighter trousers. I could fit into a dinner jacket I hadn't worn for ten years. I had also stopped snoring, which delighted my wife and quite possibly the neighbours. Even better, my blood indicators had improved in a spectacular fashion.

	MY RESULTS in mmol/l	RECOMMENDED
DIABETES RISK: FASTING GLUCOSE	5.0	3.9–5.8
HEART DISEASE FACTORS: TRIGLYCERIDES HDL CHOLESTEROL LDL CHOLESTEROL	0.6 2.1 3.6	Less than 2.3 0.9–1.5 Up to 3.0
HEART DISEASE RISK HDL % of total	37%	20% and over
CANCER RISK Somatomedin-C (IGF-1)	15.9nmol/l	11.3–30.9nmol/l

My wife Clare, who is a doctor, was astonished. She regularly sees overweight patients with blood chemistry like mine had been and she said that none of the advice she gives has anything like the same effect.

For me, the particularly pleasing changes were in my fasting glucose levels and the huge drop in my IGF-1 levels, which matched the changes I had seen after doing a four-day fast.

Clare, however, felt I was losing weight too fast, that I should consolidate for a while. That is why I decided to go on a maintenance dose of fasting just one day a week. Unless it's the weekend, holidays or a special occasion, I also, regularly, skip lunch.

What has happened is that my weight has stayed steady at 12 stone and my bloods remain in good shape. I do, however, think there is room for improvement and will shortly restart a two-day regime and blog about it. If you are interested then do visit our website, www.thefastdiet. co.uk.

So, what is the best way to go about an Intermittent Fast?

Let's recap on what we've learnt. The reason for Intermittent Fasting – briefly but severely restricting the amount of calories you consume – is that by doing so you are hoping to 'fool' your body into thinking it is in a potential famine situation and that it needs to switch from go-go mode to maintenance mode.

The reason our bodies respond to fasting in this way is that we evolved at a time when feast and famine were the norm. Our bodies are designed to respond to stresses and shocks; it makes them healthier, tougher. The scientific term is hormesis – that which does not kill you makes you stronger. The benefits of fasting include:

- Weight loss

- A reduction of IGF-1, which means that you are reducing your risk of a number of age-related diseases, such as cancer

- The switching-on of countless repair genes in response to this stressor

- Giving your pancreas a rest, which will boost the effectiveness of the insulin it produces in response to elevated blood glucose. Increased insulin sensitivity will reduce your risk of obesity, diabetes, heart disease and cognitive decline

- An overall enhancement in your mood and sense of wellbeing. This may be a consequence of your brain producing increased levels of neurotrophic factor, which will hopefully make you more cheerful, which in turn should make fasting more doable

So much for the science. In the next chapter Mimi discusses what to eat and how to go about starting life as an Intermittent Faster. How do you put the theory into practice?

THE FAST DIET IN PRACTICE

There are, as we've seen, good clinical reasons to start Intermittent Fasting. Some, such as its positive effect on blood markers, should be immediately apparent; others will become manifest over time – a cognitive boost, a self-repairing physiology, a greater chance of a longer life. But perhaps the most compelling argument for many is the promise of swift and sustained weight loss, while still eating the foods you enjoy, most of the time. You may view this as incidental to the plan's other marked health benefits. Or it may be your primary objective. The fact is you will gain both. Weight loss and better health, two sides of the same page.

Michael's experience, as described in the previous chapter, will have given you an idea of what to expect. In this chapter I will reveal more detail – explaining how to start, how it will feel, how to keep going and how the central tenets of the Fast Diet can slip easily into the rhythm of your everyday life.

Now, it's over to you.

What do 500-600 calories look like?

Cutting calories to a quarter of your usual daily intake is a significant commitment, so don't be surprised if your first fast day feels like a tough gig. As you progress, the fasts will become second nature and the initial sense of deprivation will diminish, particularly if you remain aware that tomorrow is another day – another day, in fact, when you can eat as you please.

Still, however you cut it, 500 or 600 calories is no picnic; it's not even half a picnic. A large café latte can clock in at over 300 calories, more if you insist on cream, while your usual lunchtime sandwich might easily consume your entire allowance in one huge bite. So be smart. Spend your calories wisely – the Menu Plans on pages 139-161 will be useful – but it's also worth having a clear idea of favourite fast-day foods that work for you. Remember to embrace variety: differing textures, punchy flavours, colour and crunch. Together, these things will keep your mouth entertained and stop it frowning at the hardship of it all.

When to fast

Animal studies, human studies, research, experiment: as demonstrated in the previous chapter, evidence for the value of fasting is strong. But what happens when you step out of the laboratory and into real life? When and what you eat during your 'fast' is critical to the diet's success. So what's the optimal pattern?

Michael tried several different fasting regimes; the one he settled on as the most sustainable for him is a fast on two non-consecutive days each week, allowing 600 calories a day, split between breakfast and dinner. This pattern has been called, for obvious reasons, a 5:2 diet – five days off, two days on, which means that the majority of your time is spent gloriously free from calorie-counting. On a fast day, he'll normally have breakfast with the family at around 7.30am and then aim to have dinner with them at 7.30pm, with nothing eaten in between. That way, he gets two 12-hour fasts in a day, and a happy family at the end of it.

The menu suggestions on pages 139-161 are based on this pattern as it is, in his experience, the most straightforward Intermittent Fasting method.

As will become clear later in this chapter, I found that a slightly different pattern works for me. Sticking to the Fast Diet's central tenet, I eat 500 calories – but as two meals with a few snacks (an apple, some carrot sticks) in between, simply because the vast plain between breakfast and supper feels too great, too empty for comfort. There is evidence, from trials conducted by Dr Michelle Harvie[17] and others, that this approach will help you lose weight, reduce your risk of breast cancer and increase insulin sensitivity.

Which approach is better? At this point, given that the science of Intermittent Fasting is still in its infancy, we don't know. On purely theoretical grounds, a longer period without food (Michael's pattern) might be expected to produce better results than one where you eat smaller amounts more frequently. But as far as we are aware there have, as yet, been no studies which attempt to compare the health benefits to people on a fasting day of either eating their calories in one go, split up or spread throughout the day. When we know more we will update you.

Professor Mark Mattson at the National Institute on Aging says that by eating your calories as a single meal you might get a modestly greater ketogenic ('fat-burning') effect, compared to three very small meals spread through the day. But he also thinks we shouldn't get too hung up about it. 'Regardless of whether the 600 calories is consumed as one meal or two or three smaller meals, you will get major health benefits.'

We await more trials but it is already clear from the hundreds who have tried it that as long as you stick to the Fast Diet you will enjoy that crucial combination of weight loss, health benefits and cheerful compliance.

Some people who don't feel hungry at breakfast would rather eat later in the day. That's fine. One of the key researchers in this field often starts her day with a late breakfast at around 11am and finishes with supper at 7pm. That way, she's fasting for 16 hours a day, twice a week. Based on the mouse study cited on page 28, it may even be a better approach.

It is, however, only better if you actually do it, and a delayed breakfast may not suit some lifestyles, timetables or bodies. So go with a timetable that suits you. Some fasters will appreciate the convenience and simplicity of a single 500- or 600-calorie meal, allowing them to ignore food entirely for most of the day. Whatever you choose, it must be your plan, your life. Do it with gusto, but be prepared to experiment, within the limits set out by the plan.

What to eat

It may seem curious to talk about what to eat when you are fasting. But the Fast Diet is a modified programme, allowing 500 calories for a woman and 600 for a man on any given fast day, making the regime relatively comfortable and, above all, sustainable over the longterm. So, yes, you do get to eat on a fast day. But it matters what you choose.

There are two general principles that should govern what you eat and what you avoid on a fast day. Your aim is to have food that makes you feel satisfied, but stays firmly within the 500/600 calorie allowance – and the best options to achieve this are foods that are high in protein, and foods with a low glycaemic index (GI).

There have been a number of studies demonstrating that individuals who eat a diet higher in protein feel fuller for longer (indeed the main reason why people lose weight on diets like Atkins is because they eat less).[18] The trouble with really high-protein diets, however, is that people tend to get bored of the food restrictions and give up.

There is also evidence that high-protein diets are associated with higher levels of chronic inflammation and IGF-1, which in turn are associated with increased risk of heart disease and cancer.[19]

So the Fast Diet does not recommend boycotting carbs entirely, or living permanently on a high-protein diet. However, on a fast day, the combination of proteins and foods with a low GI will be helpful weapons in keeping hunger at bay.

Understanding the glycaemic index

In earlier chapters, we discovered the importance of blood sugar and insulin. High levels of insulin brought about by high levels of blood sugar will encourage your body to store fat and increase your cancer risk. Another reason not to eat foods that make your blood sugar levels surge, particularly on your fast days, is that when your blood sugar crashes, as it inevitably will, you will start feeling very hungry indeed.

Carbohydrates have the biggest impact on blood

sugars, but not all carbs are equal. As habitual dieters will know, one way to discover which carbs cause a big spike and which don't is to look at their GI. Each food gets a score out of 100, with a low score meaning that the particular food does not tend to cause a rapid rise in blood glucose. These are the ones you want.

The size of the sugar spike depends both on the food itself, and on how much of it you eat. For example, we tend to eat a lot more potatoes in one sitting than kiwi fruit. So there's also a measure called GL, the Glycaemic Load, which:

$$\frac{GI \times grams\ of\ carbohydrate}{100}$$

This makes some pretty heroic assumptions about the amount of a particular food you are likely to eat as a portion, but at least it is a guide.

The reason GI and GL are interesting is not just because they are strongly predictive of future health (people on a low GL diet have less risk of diabetes, heart disease and various cancers), but because there are so many surprises. Who would have imagined that eating a baked potato would have as big an impact on your blood glucose as eating a tablespoon of sugar?

Broadly speaking a GI over 50 or a GL over 20 is not good, and the lower both figures are the better. It is worth restating that GI and GL are measures that relate to carbs.

GI is not relevant to protein and fats, which is why none of the foods listed have a significant protein or fat content. As an example, let's take a quick look at breakfast:

BREAKFAST	GI	GL
PORRIDGE	50	10
MUESLI	50	10
BAGUETTE	95	15
CROISSANT	67	17
CORNFLAKES	80	20

Source: http://people.bu.edu/sobieraj/papers/GlycemicIndices.pdf

You can see why, if you are having a carb breakfast, porridge and muesli are better options than cornflakes or a croissant. And what are you going to put on your muesli?

	GI	GL
MILK	27	3
SOY MILK	44	8

The relatively high GI and GL of soy milk is just one reason to stick with dairy. And since we're handing out surprises, here's another one:

	GI	GL
ICE CREAM	37	4

You would bet your house on ice cream being high GI/GL, but not so. If you factor it into your calorie count, low-calorie ice cream with strawberries is a treat to round off a meal. For more on the GI and GL of various foods and how best to plan your fast-day foods, see pages 107-8.

What about protein?

We certainly don't recommend eating protein to the exclusion of all else on a fast day, but you do require an adequate quantity, for muscle health, cell maintenance, endocrinal regulation, immunity and energy. Protein is satiating too, so it's well worth including it in your calorie quota. While Valter Longo recommends 0.8g of protein per kg of body weight per day – which would give a 12 stone man around 60g, and a nine-stone woman around 45g – perhaps the simplest method is to stick to recommended governmental guidelines, which allow for a (quite generous) 50g per day.

Go for 'good protein'. Steamed white fish, for example, is low in saturated fats and rich in minerals. Choose skinless chicken over red meat; try low-fat dairy products over endless lattes; include prawns, tuna, tofu and other plant proteins. Nuts, seeds, pulses and legumes are full of fibre and act as bulking agents on a hungry day. Nuts – though high in calories (depending, of course, on how many you eat) – are generally low GI and brilliantly satiating. They are fatty too, so you might imagine they are 'bad for you', yet the evidence is that nut consumers have lower rates of heart disease and diabetes than nut abstainers.[20]

Eggs, meanwhile, are low in saturated fat and full of nutritional value; they won't adversely affect your cholesterol levels and they score a mere 85 calories each, so an egg-based breakfast on a fast day makes perfect sense. Two eggs plus a 50g serving of smoked salmon clocks in at a sensible 250 calories. Research recently found that individuals who consume egg protein for breakfast are more likely to feel full during the day than those whose breakfasts contain wheat protein.[21] Poaching or boiling an egg avoids the addition of careless calories. Stand down the toast soldiers and replace with steamed asparagus spears. For more suggestions about foods to keep you full and fit on a fast day, and the benefits certain choices will bring, turn to page 107-8.

How to fit fasting into your life

When to start?

If you do not have an underlying medical condition, and if you are not an individual for whom fasting is proscribed (see pages 123-4), then there really is no time like the present. Ask yourself: if not now, when? You may prefer to await a doctor's advice. You may choose to prepare yourself, talk yourself down from a lifelong habit of overeating, clear out the fridge, eat the last cookie in the jar, have a scratch. Or you may want to get on with it and start to see visible progress within a couple of weeks. Do, however, begin on a day when you feel strong, purposeful, calm and committed. Do tell friends and family that you're starting the Fast Diet: once you make a public commitment, you are much more likely to stick with it. Avoid high days, holidays and days when you're booked in for a three-course lunch complete with bread basket, cheese board and four types of dessert. Recognise, too, that a busy day will help your fast time fly, while a duvet day generally crawls by like honey off a spoon. Once you've deliberated and designated a day to debut, get your mind in gear. Record your details – weight, BMI, target – before you start and note your progress in a diary, knowing that dieters who keep an honest account of what they eat and drink are more likely to lose the pounds and keep them off. Then… take a deep breath and relax. Better yet, shrug. It's no big deal: you have nothing to lose but weight.

How tough will it be?

If it has been a while since you have experienced hunger, even the slightest hint, you'll probably find that eating no more than 500 or 600 calories in a day is a mild challenge, at least initially. Intermittent Fasters do report that the process becomes significantly easier with time, particularly as they witness results in the mirror and on the scales. Your first fast day should speed by, buoyed along by the novelty of the process; a fast day on a wet Wednesday in week three may feel more of a slog.

Your mission is to complete it, knowing that, although you are saying no to chocolate today, you will be eating what you want tomorrow. That is the joy of the Fast Diet and what makes it so different from other weight-loss plans.

How to win the hunger games

There is no reason to be alarmed by benign, occasional, short-term hunger. Given base-level good health, you will not perish. You won't collapse in a heap and need to be rescued by the cat. Your body is designed to go without food for longish periods, even if it has lost the skill through years of grazing, picking and snacking. Research has found that modern humans tend to mistake a whole range of emotions for hunger.[22] We eat when we're bored, when we're thirsty, when we're around food (when aren't we?), when we're in company or simply when the clock happens to tell us it's time for food. Most of us eat, too, just because it feels good. This is known as 'hedonic hunger' – and while you should try to resist it on a fast day, you can bask in the knowledge that, if you please, you can give in to temptation the following day.

There's no need to panic about any of this. Simply note that the human brain is adept at persuading us that we're hungry in almost all situations: when faced with feelings of deprivation or withdrawal or disappointment; when angry, sad, happy, neutral; when subject to advertising, social imperatives, sensory stimulation, reward, habit, the smell of freshly brewed coffee or baking bread or bacon cooking in a café up the road. Recognise now that these are often learnt reactions to external cues, most of them designed to part you from your cash. If you are still processing your last meal, it's highly unlikely that what you are experiencing is true hunger ('total transit time', should you be interested in such things, can take up to two days, depending on your gender, your metabolism and what you've eaten).

While hunger pangs can be aggressive and disagreeable, like a box of sharp knives, in practice, they are more fluid and controllable than you might think. You're unlikely to be troubled at all by hunger until well into a fast day. What's more, a pang will pass. Fasters report that the feeling of perceived hunger comes in waves, not in an ever-growing wall of gnawing belly noise. It's a symphony of differentiated movements, not a steady, fearful crescendo. Treat a tummy rumble as a good sign, a healthy messenger.

Remember, too, that hunger does not build over a 24-hour period, so don't feel trapped in the feeling at any given moment.

Wait a while. You have absolute power to conquer feelings of hunger, simply by steering your mind, riding the wave, choosing to do something else – take a walk, phone a friend, drink tea, go for a run, take a shower, sing in the shower, phone a friend from the shower and sing… After a few weeks' practising Intermittent Fasting, people generally report that their sense of hunger is diminished.

The main struggle with doing the Fast Diet or any form of fasting is the first few weeks while your body and mind adjust to new habits, new ways of eating. The good news is that most people find they soon adapt. In fact many people have contacted us to say that it is unexpectedly easy.

Kimberley, who has been following the 5:2 method with her husband for some time, says: 'I am amazed at the energy I have during the Fast Days. It is not terribly difficult but is mildly challenging. I've done Weight Watchers over and over and this is so much easier. Many of my friends are interested to see how we do. So far, I feel like my belly has gone down. My hubby's blood pressure is down 10+ points, systolic and diastolic.'

The important thing is to have a strategy that works for you. David, for example, wrote, 'I find even a small breakfast triggers hunger for the rest of the day, so I avoid eating anything until late on. You have to approach a Fast Day in the right mindset.'

So, take heart. On a Fast Day, refrain, restrain, divert and distract. Before you know it, you've retrained your brain and hunger's off the menu.

Tomorrow is another day: will power, patience and delayed gratification

Perhaps the most reassuring, and game-changing, part of the Fast Diet is that it doesn't last for ever. Unlike deprivation diets that have failed you before, on this plan, tomorrow will always be different. Easier. There may be pancakes for breakfast, or lunch with friends, wine with supper, apple pie with cream.

This On/Off switch is critical. It means that, on a fast day, though you're eating a quarter of your usual calorie intake, tomorrow you can eat as you please. There's boundless psychological comfort in the fact that your fasting will only ever be a short stay, a brief break from food.

When you're not fasting, ignore fasting – it doesn't own you, it doesn't define you. You're not even doing it most of the time. Unlike full-time fad diets, you'll still get pleasure from food, you'll still have treats, you'll engage in the regular, routine, food-related events of your normal life. There are no special shakes, bars, rules, points, affectations or idiosyncrasies. No saying 'no' all the time.

For this reason, you won't feel serially deprived – which, as anyone who has embarked on the grinding chore of long-term every-day dieting, the kind that makes you want to commit hara-kiri right there on the kitchen floor every time you open the fridge door, is precisely why conventional diet plans fail.

The key, then, is to recognise, through patience and the exercise of will, that you can make it through to breakfast. Bear in mind that fasting subjects regularly report that the food with which they 'break their fast' tastes glorious. Flavours sing. Mouthfuls dance. If you've ever felt a lazy disregard for the food you consume without thinking, then things are about to change. There's nothing like a bit of delayed gratification to make things taste good.

Compliance and sustainability: how to discover a sensible eating pattern that works for you

Most diets don't work. You know that already. Indeed, when a team of psychologists at UCLA conducted an analysis of 31 long-term diet trials back in 2007, they concluded that 'several studies indicate that dieting is a consistent predictor of future weight gain… We asked what evidence there is that dieting works in the long term, and found that the evidence shows the opposite.' Their analysis found that, while slimmers do lose pounds in the early months, the vast majority return to their original weight within five years, while 'at least a third end up heavier than when they embarked on the project'.[23] The standard approach clearly hasn't worked, doesn't work and won't work.

In order to be effective, then, any method must be rational, sustainable, flexible and feasible for the long haul. Adherence, not weight loss per se, is the key, so your goals must be realistic and the programme practical. It must fit into your life as it is, not the life of your dreams. It needs to go on holiday with you, it needs to visit friends, get you through a boring day at the office and cope with Christmas. To work at all, any weight-loss strategy has to be tolerable, organic and innate, not some spurious add-on that makes you feel awkward and self-conscious, the dietary equivalent of uncomfortable shoes.

While the long-term experience of Intermittent Fasters is still under investigation, people who have tried it comment on how easily it fits into everyday life. They still get variety from food (anyone who's ever tried to lose weight on 'only' grapefruit or cabbage soup will know how vital this is). They still get rewards from food. They still get a life. There is no drama, no desperate dieting, no self-flagellation. No sweat.

Flexibility: your key to success

Your body is not my body. Mine is not yours. So it's worth carving out your plan according to your needs, the shape of your day, your family, your commitments, your preferences. We none of us live cookie-cutter lives, and no single diet plan fits all. Everyone has quirks and qualifiers. That's why there are no absolute commandments here, just suggestions. You may choose to fast in a particular way, on a particular day. You may like to eat once, or twice, first thing or last. You may like beetroot or fennel or blueberries.

Some individuals prefer to be told exactly what to eat and when; others like a more informal approach. That's fine. It's enough to simply stick to the basic method – 500 or 600 calories a day, with as long a window without food as possible, twice a week – and you'll gain the plan's multiple benefits. In time, there's little need for assiduous calorie counting; you'll know what a fast day means and how to make it suit you.

The Maintenance Model

Once you've reached your target weight, or just a shade below (allowing room for manoeuvre and a generous slice of birthday cake), you may consider adopting the Maintenance Model. This is an adjustment to fasting on only one day each week in order to remain in a holding pattern at your desired weight, but still reap the benefits of occasional fasting.

Naturally, one day a week – if that's what you choose – may offer fewer health benefits than two in the long run; but it does fit neatly into a life, particularly if you are not intent on achieving any further weight loss.

Equally, if the beach beckons or there's a wedding in the diary or you've woken up on Boxing Day haunted by that fourth roast potato, step it up again. You're in charge.

What to expect

The first thing you can expect from adopting the Fast Diet, of course, is to lose weight: some weeks more, some weeks less; some weeks finding yourself stuck at a disappointing plateau, other weeks making swifter progress. As a basic guide, you might anticipate a loss of around a pound with each fast day. This will not, of course, be all fat. Some will be water, and the digested food in your system. You should, however, lose around ten pounds of fat over a ten-week period, which beats a typical low-calorie diet. Crucially, you can expect to maintain your weight loss over time.

More important than what you'll lose, though, is what you're set to gain…

How your anatomy will change

Over a period of weeks, you can expect your BMI, your levels of body fat and your waist measurement to gradually fall. Your cholesterol and triglyceride levels should also improve. This is the path to greater health and extended life. You are already dodging your unwritten future. Right now, though, the palpable changes will start to show up in the mirror as your body becomes leaner and lighter.

As the weeks progress, you'll find that Intermittent Fasting has potent secondary effects too. Alongside the obvious weight loss and the health benefits stored up for the future, there are more subtle consequences, perks and bonuses that can come into play.

How your appetite will change

Expect your food preferences to adapt; pretty soon, you'll start to choose healthy foods by default rather than by design. You will begin to understand hunger, to negotiate and manage it, knowing how it feels to be properly hungry; you'll also recognise the sensation of being pleasantly full, not groaning like an immovable sofa. Satiated, not stuffed. The upshot? No more 'food hangovers', improved digestion, more bounce.

After six months of Intermittent Fasting, interesting things should happen to your eating habits. You may find that you eat half the meat you once did – not as a conscious move, but as a natural one born of what you desire rather than what you decide or believe. You're likely to consume more veg. Many Intermittent Fasters instinctively retreat from bread (and, by association, butter), while stodgy 'comfort' foods seem less appealing and refined sugars aren't nearly as tempting as they once were. The bag of Haribo in the glove box of the car? Take it or leave it.

Of course, you don't need to dwell actively on any of this. It will happen anyway. If you are like me, then one day soon, you'll arrive at a place where you say no to the cheesecake because you don't fancy it, not because you are denying yourself a treat.

This is the baseline power of Intermittent Fasting: it encourages you to recheck your diet. And that's your long-haul ticket to health.

How your attitude will change

So, yes, you'll start to lose bad habits around food. But if you continue to fast – and feast – with awareness, all kinds of other changes should occur, some of them unlikely and unexpected.

You may, for instance, discover that you've been suffering from 'portion distortion' for years, thinking that the food piled on your plate is the quantity you really need and want. With time, you'll probably discover that you've been overdoing it. Muffins will start to look vast as they sit, fat and moist, under glass domes in coffee shops. A maxi bag of crisps becomes a monstrous prospect. You may go from Venti to Grande to wanting only half a cup, no sugar, no cream.

Soon, you'll come to recognise the truth about how you've been eating and the wordless fibs you've told yourself for years. This is as much a part of the recalibrating process as anything else; you've changed your mind. Occasional fasting will train you in the art of 'restrained eating'; in the last instance, this is the goal. It's all part of the long game of behavioural change that means that the Fast Diet will ultimately become neither a fast, nor a diet, but a way of life.

After a while, you'll have cultivated a new approach to eating – thoughtful, rational, responsible – without even knowing you're doing it.

Intermittent Fasters also report a boost in their energy, together with an amplified sense of emotional wellbeing. Some talk of a 'glow' – the result, perhaps, of winning the battle for self-control, or of the smaller clothes and the compliments, or of something going on at a metabolic level that governs our moods. We may not yet know precisely why, but whatever it is, it feels good. Far better than cake. As one online devotee says, 'Overall, fasting just seems right. It's like a reset button for your entire body.'[24]

More subtly still, many fasters acknowledge a sense of relief as their fast days no longer revolve around food. Embrace it. There's a certain liberty here, if you allow it to materialise. You may find, as we have, that you start to look forward to your fasts: a time to regroup and give feeding a rest.

The Fast Diet in reality: tales, tips and troubleshooting

How men fast: Michael's experience

A lot of men have contacted me over the last few months to let me know how much weight they have lost and also to say how surprised and delighted they are that Intermittent Fasting turns out to be so easy. They like its simplicity, the fact that you don't have to give things up or try to remember complicated recipes. I also think they rather like the challenge.

The actor and comedian Dom Joly recently wrote that he'd lost two and a half stone after watching my *Horizon* programme and felt it was an approach he could imagine sticking to for the rest of his life.[25] The attraction for him is that he knows he will be able to eat what he wants the following day. He even added that he now rather enjoys the fasting days, something I have heard from a number of men. One of the things that men seem to like particularly about fasting is that they can fit it into their lives with minimal hassle. It doesn't stop them working, travelling, socialising or exercising. In fact, some find it fuels performance (see page 121 for more on fasting and exercise).

In one Belgian study, men asked to eat a high-fat diet and exercise before breakfast on an empty stomach put on far less weight than a similar group of men on an identical diet who exercised after breakfast.[26] This study adds support to the claim that exercising in a fasted state makes the body burn a greater percentage of fat for fuel. At least it does if you are a man.

For me, a fast day now follows a familiar routine. I start with a protein-rich breakfast, normally scrambled eggs or kippers. I drink several cups of black coffee and tea during the day, work happily through lunch and rarely feel any hunger pangs until well into the late afternoon. When they happen, I simply ignore them or go for a brief stroll until they pass.

In the evening I have a bit of meat or fish and piles of steamed vegetables. Having abstained since breakfast I find them particularly delicious.

I never have problems getting to sleep and most days wake up the next morning feeling no more peckish than normal.

How women fast: Mimi's experience

While most men I know respond well to numbers and targets (with associated gadgets if at all possible), I've found that women tend to take a more holistic approach to fasting. As with much in life, we like to examine how it feels, knowing that our bodies are unique and will respond to any given stimulation in their own sweet way. We respond to shared stories and the support of friends. And, sometimes, we need a snack.

Personally, for instance, I like to consume my fast-day calories in two lots, one early, one late, bookending the day with my allowance and aiming for a longish gap in between to maximise the prospect of health gains and weight loss. But I do need a little something to keep me going in between. A fast-day breakfast is usually a low-sugar muesli, perhaps including some fresh strawberries and almonds, with semi-skimmed milk; there'll be an apple 'for lunch' – hardly a feast, I know, but just enough to make a difference to the day. Then, supper: a substantial, interesting salad with heaps of leaves and some lean protein – perhaps smoked salmon or tuna or hummus – once the kids are in bed. Throughout the day, I drink San Pellegrino mineral water with a squeeze of lime, tons of herbal tea and plenty of black coffee. They just help the day tick by.

In the four months since I started the Fast Diet, I have lost 6kg, and my BMI has gone from 21.4 to 19.4. If you're struggling with bigger numbers than these, take strength from the fact that heavier subjects respond brilliantly to Intermittent Fasting, and the positive effects should be apparent in a relatively short time. These days, one fast a week (on Mondays) seems to suffice and keep me at a stable, happy weight.

Many women I encounter are well versed in dieting techniques (years of practice), and I've found that a couple of tips can come in handy on a fast day. I'd recommend, for instance, eating in small mouthfuls, chewing slowly and concentrating when eating. Why read a magazine, why tweet as you eat? If you're only getting 500 calories, it makes sense to notice them as they go in.

I have found, like many Intermittent Fasters, that hunger is simply not an issue. For whatever reason – and one wonders whether it suits the food industry – we have developed a fear of hunger, fretting about low blood sugar and whatnot.

On the whole, for me, a day with little food feels emancipating rather than restrictive. That said, there are ups and downs: some days skim by like a stone on water; other days, I feel like I'm sinking, not swimming, perhaps because emotions or hormones or simply the tricky business of life have kicked in. See how you feel, and always give in gracefully if that particular day is not your day to fast.

A dozen ways to make the Fast Diet work for you

1. *Know your weight, your BMI and your waist size from the get-go.* As we mentioned earlier, waist measurement is a simple and important measurement of internal fat and a powerful predictor of future health. People who do Intermittent Fasting soon lose those dangerous and unattractive inches. BMI is your weight (in kilograms) divided by your height (in metres) squared; it may sound like a palaver, and an abstract one at that, but it's a widely accepted tool for plotting a path to healthy weight loss. Do note that a BMI score takes no account of body type, age or ethnicity, so should be greeted with informed caution. Still, if you need a number, this is a useful one.

Weigh yourself regularly but not obsessively. After the initial stages, once a week should suffice. The mornings after fast days are best if you like to see falling figures. You may discover that your weight measurement is significantly different from feed day to Fast Day. This discrepancy may well be due to the additional weight of food in your system, rather than changes in your fat mass from one day to the next. You may like to take an average over several days to arrive at a reasonable figure for any weight loss. But don't overdo it; try not to make weighing – yourself or your calories – a chore.

If you are someone who enjoys structure and clarity, you may want to monitor your progress. Have a target in mind. Where do you want to be, and when? Be realistic:

precipitous weight loss is not advised, so allow yourself time. Make a plan. Write it down.

Plenty of people recommend keeping a diet diary. Alongside the numbers, add your experiences; try to note down three good things that happen on each day. It's a feel-good message that you can refer to as time goes by.

2. *Find a fast friend.* You need very few accoutrements to make this a success, but a supportive friend may well be one of them. Once you're on the Fast Diet, tell people about it; you may find that they join in, and you'll develop a network of common experience. Since the plan appeals to men and women equally, couples report that they find it more manageable to do it together. That way, you get mutual support, camaraderie, joint commitment and shared anecdotes; besides, meal times are made infinitely easier if you're eating with someone who understands the rudiments of the plot. There are plenty of threads on online chat rooms too. Mumsnet is a great source of support and information. It's remarkable how reassuring it is to know that you're not alone.

3. *Prep your fast-day food in advance* so that you don't go foraging and come across a leftover sausage lurking irresistibly in the fridge. Keep it simple, aiming for fast-day flavour without effort. Shop and cook on non-fast days, so as not to taunt yourself with undue temptation

(For simple, sustaining fast-day recipe ideas, see pages 139-61). Before you embark, clear the house of junk food. It will only croon and coo at you from the cupboards, making your fast day harder than it needs to be.

4. *Check calorie labels for portion size.* When the cereal box says 'a 30g serving', measure it. Go on. Be amazed. Then be honest. Since your calorie count on a fast day is necessarily fixed and limited, it's important not to be blinkered about how much is actually going in. You'll find a calorie counter for suggested fast-day foods on page 185. Or download a calorie counter app such as www.myfitnesspal.com. Nutratech.co.uk offers a useful online interactive food diary – go to www.nutratech.co.uk. Alternatively, www.nutritiondata.self.com includes specific search criteria to allow you to match your food choices not only to your calorie allocation but also to your nutritional needs. Way more importantly, don't count calories on a non-fast day. You've got better things to do.

5. *Wait before you eat.* Try to resist for at least ten minutes, 15 if you can, to see if the hunger subsides (as it naturally tends to do). If you absolutely must snack, choose something that will not elevate your insulin levels. Try some julienned carrots, a handful of plain air-popped popcorn, an apple slice or some strawberries. But don't pick and peck like a hen through the day; the calories will soon stack up and your fast will be dashed. On fast days, eat with awareness, allowing yourself to fully absorb the fact that you're eating (not as daft as it sounds, particularly if you have ever sat in a traffic jam popping M&Ms). Similarly, on off-duty days, stay gently alert. Eat until you're satisfied, not until you're full (this will come naturally after a few weeks' practice). Work out what the concept of 'fullness' means for you – we are all different and it changes over time.

6. *Stay busy.* 'We humans are always looking for things to do between meals,' said Leonard Cohen. Yes, and look where it's got us. So fill your day, not your face. As fasting advocate Brad Pilon has noted, 'No one's hungry in the first few seconds of a sky dive.' Engage in things other than food – not necessarily sky diving, but anything that appeals to you. Distraction is your best defence against the dark arts of the food industry, which has stationed donuts on every street corner and nachos at every turn. And remember, if you must have that donut, it will still be there tomorrow.

7. *Try the two-to-two*: fasting not from bedtime to bedtime, but from 2pm until 2pm. After lunch on day one, eat sparingly until a late lunch the following day. That way, you lose weight as you sleep and no single day feels uncomfortably deprived of food. It's a clever trick, but it does require a modicum more concentration than the whole-day option. Or perhaps fast from supper to supper, which again means that no day is All Fast and No Fun. The point is that this plan is 'adjust to fit'. Just like your waistband in three weeks' time…

8. *Don't be afraid to think about food you like.* A psychological mechanism called 'habituation' – in which the more people have of something, the less value they attach to it – means that doing the opposite and trying to suppress thoughts of food is a 'flawed strategy'.[27] The critical thought process here is to treat food as a friend, not as a foe. Food is not magical, supernatural or dangerous. Don't demonise it; normalise it. It's only food.

9. *Stay hydrated.* Find no-calorie drinks you like, and then drink them in quantity. Some swear by herbal tea; others prefer a mineral water with bubbles to dance on the tongue, though tap water will do just as well. Plenty of our hydration comes through the food we eat, so you may need to compensate with additional drinks beyond your routine intake (check your urine; it should be plentiful and pale). While there's no scientific rationale for drinking the recommended eight glasses of water a day, there is good reason to keep the liquids coming in. A dry mouth is the last sign of dehydration, not the first, so act before your body complains, recognising too that a glass of water is a quick way to hush an empty belly, at least temporarily. It will also stop you mistaking thirst for hunger.

10. *Don't count on weight loss on any given day.* If you have a week when the scales don't seem to shift, dwell instead upon the health benefits you will certainly be accruing even if you haven't seen your numbers drop. Remember why you're doing this: not just the smaller jeans, but the longterm advantages, the widely accepted disease-busting, brain-boosting, life-lengthening benefits of Intermittent Fasting. Think of it as a pension plan for your body.

11. *Be sensible, exercise caution, and if it feels wrong, stop.* It's vital that this strategy should be practised in a way that's flexible and forgiving. It's OK to break the rules if you need to. It's not a race to the finish, so be kind to yourself and make it fun. Who wants to live longer if life's an abject misery? You don't want to grunt and sweat under a weary life. You want to go dancing. Right?

12. *Congratulate yourself.* Every completed fast day means potential weight loss and quantifiable health gain. You're already winning.

Q & A

Which days should I choose to fast?
It really doesn't matter. It's your life, and you'll know which days will suit you best. Monday is an obvious choice for many, perhaps because it is more manageable,

psychologically and practically, to gear yourself up at the beginning of a new week, particularly if it follows a sociable weekend. For that reason, fasters might choose to avoid Saturdays and Sundays, when family lunches and brunches, dinner dates and parties make calorie-cutting a chore. Thursday would then make a sensible second fasting day, chiming, if such things appeal, with the teachings of the Prophet Mohammed, who is understood to have fasted on the second and fifth days of the week. But be flexible; don't force yourself to fast when it feels wrong. If you're particularly stressed, off-colour, tired or peevish on a day that you have designated a fast, try again another day. Adapt. This is not about one-size-fits-all rules; it's about finding a realistic pattern that works for you. Do, however, aim for a pattern. That way, over time, your fasts will become familiar, a low-key habit you accept and embrace. You may adapt your fasts as your life (and your body) changes shape – but don't drop too many fast days; there is a danger that you'll slide back into old habits. Be kind. But be tough.

Does it have to be for 24 hours?

Fasting for a 24-hour period is practical, coherent and unambiguous, all of which will promise a greater chance of success. It is, however, merely the most convenient way of organising a fast: there's nothing magical about 24 hours. To save on bother, stick to it, and remind yourself that you'll be asleep for nearly a third of it.

Should I fast on consecutive days?

Many of the studies done to date on humans have involved volunteers fasting on consecutive days; there is certainly value in doing back-to-back fasts, but as far as we are aware, there are no studies on humans comparing this approach with split days. We do, however, know what works in practice for fasters like us. Michael tried the consecutive system and found it too challenging to be sustainable over time, so he switched to the split version – fasting on Mondays and Thursdays. The weight loss, improvements in glucose, cholesterol and IGF-1 that he saw are all based on this non-consecutive, two-day pattern.

There's a psychological imperative here too: fast for more than a day at a time, and you may start to feel resentful, bored and beleaguered – precisely the feelings that wreck the best-made diet intentions. A critical part of this plan is that you never feel challenged for long enough to consider quitting. By the time you've had enough, breakfast is on the table and another fast has passed.

How much weight will I lose?

This will depend largely on your own metabolism, your individual body type, your starting weight, your level of activity and how effectively and honestly you fast. In the first week, you may experience water loss that can account for a significant dip on the scales; with time, your weekly calorie deficit will mean, thanks to the simple law of thermogenics (energy in < energy out = weight loss), that you will be losing fat. Be judicious: abrupt weight loss is not advised and shouldn't be your aim. You may, however, anticipate losing around half a stone in eight weeks.

I know I should stick to low GI foods on a fast day. So which foods are best?

As we've seen, foods with a low GI or GL will help keep your blood sugar stable, increasing your chances of a successful day with few calories. Vegetables and legumes are, needless to say, amazing, and you should rely on them on a fast day. Packed with nutrients, their bulk fills you up, they have relatively few calories and they keep your blood sugar low. Carrots are a great snack, particularly with hummus dip, which scores an astonishing GI of 6 and a GL of 0. Fruit is handy too, though some fruits are more fast-friendly than others.

Check the GI count of your chosen fast-day foods online. Diabetes UK has an excellent guide at www.diabetes.org.uk.

Or look at the GI Index from the University of Sydney on www.glycemicindex.com, noting that some foods have an unexpected count. Staples, for instance, are worth scrutinising with an eagle eye:

STAPLES	GI	GL
BROWN RICE	48	20
WHITE RICE	76	36

	GI	GL
PASTA durum wheat	40	20
COUSCOUS	65	23
POTATOES BOILED	58	16
MASHED	85	17
FRIED	75	22
BAKED	85	26

The biggest surprise regarding the staples is how big an effect baking or mashing potatoes has on blood sugars. On fast days, avoid these starchy basics, and substitute with plenty of greens. Fill your plate. Watch out for fruit too. Some are your fast friends; others will spike your blood sugar and are best left for the days when you are eating freely.

FRUIT	GI	GL
STRAWBERRIES	38	1
APPLES	35	5
ORANGES	42	5
GRAPES	45	9
PINEAPPLE	84	7
BANANAS	50	12
RAISINS	64	30
DATES	100	42

Eating the whole fruit will keep you feeling full for longer.

Strawberries, without sugar, are extraordinarily low GI/GL and also low calorie (no wonder many fasters eat a bowl for breakfast). The striking thing to note is the high sugar impact of raisins and dates. Avoid them on fast days. For more on calorie levels, refer to the Counter on page 185.

I've read about 'super-foods' and 'intelligent eating'. Should I include super-foods during a fast day?

The term 'super-food' is more of a marketing ploy than a scientific construct, and clinical nutritionists are loath to use the description. All plants produce a huge range of phytochemicals that can have a beneficial role in the body: eat them on a fast day or, indeed, on any day you please. The following foods taste good and they're generally low in calories – making them ideal fast-day companions:

- **FRUIT:** As the labs of the world continue in their quest for new anti-obesity marvels, the latest to emerge is the humble tangerine. Citrus fruits in general, and tangerines in particular, contain high concentrations of nobiletin, a compound that 'protects from obesity and atherosclerosis' – in lab mice at least.[28] If you like tangerines, eat them, perhaps spending time meditatively peeling away the pith. The same group of researchers previously found that grapefruit, rich in a compound called naringenin, encourages the liver to burn fat rather than store it.[29] Grapefruit also contains compounds such as liminoids and lycopene (thought to have anti-cancer properties),[30] and clocks in at only 39 calories per half, making it a good fast-day food. (You should, however, be aware that grapefruit interacts with a number of common medicines, so if you are taking medication such as statins, consult your doctor.) Alternatively, you could always throw in a watermelon smile (30 calories per 100g) or an apple (around 50 calories per 100g) for flavour, crunch and pectin, a soluble fibre that can't be absorbed by the body but is useful in fat digestion.[31] Apples are the ultimate convenience food, though they are quite high in calories; eat the whole thing, skin, pips and core – you'll probably want to if it's one of your fast day treats. Tomatoes also contain lycopene, which may help guard against cancer[32] and stroke.[33] A handful of cherry tomatoes or strawberries (low GI, low GL) could be your best bet to get you through a tummy rumble unscathed. Check for calorie traps before you eat (see the Calorie Counter on page 185)

- **BERRIES:** Blueberries are high in antioxidant polyphenols and phytonutrients. New research has found that these bold little berries may also be able to break down fat cells in the body and prevent new ones from forming.[34] Pretty impressive, eh? Even if you don't buy the science, blueberries remain a handy source of vitamin C. Once you're berry savvy, you may want to cruise your local healthfood store for other super-foods: goji, acai, aloe, hemp seeds, chia seeds and spirulina (a nutrient-rich blue-green alga). All curious, all good

- **VEGETABLES:** Again, aim for a broad variety – different colours, textures, tastes, shapes. Steamed broccoli contains a whole world of nutrients (including vitamin K). Green beans love a little lemon and garlic. Fennel is great if shaved (invest in a mandolin), perhaps teamed with orange segments and a squeeze of the juice. Edamame are a good source of low-fat protein and omega 3 fatty acids. Starchy veg, of course, tend to have a higher GL and calorific value, though they are satiating. Proceed with caution and don't add butter

- **LEAVES:** It goes without saying that green leafy veg are your fast-day friends. Spinach, kale, chard, mustard greens, salad leaves… a veritable vit fest, and agreeably low in calories. Pep things up with chilli flakes, ginger, cumin, pepper, lemon juice, garlic. Garlic, by the way, contains allicin, the active ingredient that lends it pungency and is also thought to protect cells and reduce fatty deposits,[35] so be liberal and carry (sugarless) mints

- **HERBS AND SPICES:** Low-cal, high-impact, no brainer. Pickles may work for you too – cornichons, jalapenos, onions (watch the GI values) – or mustard; anything, really, that brings a bolt of fire or flavour to your plate

- **NUTS:** We've established that nuts are a fast-day favourite: filling and low GI. Almonds, though calorific, are high in protein and fibre which makes them brilliantly satiating; pistachios too (better yet, they take ages to crack and eat). Cashews and coconut flakes will help animate a salad. But count wisely: nut calories soon clock up

- **SEEDS:** Sunflower seeds contain good fats, together with iron, zinc, potassium, vitamins E and B1, magnesium and selenium – all that goodness in a tiny little packet

- **SOUP:** Scientists at Penn State University have found that soup is a great appetite suppressant.[36] Go for a light broth, a miso soup, a kicky pho; choose carrot and coriander over a creamy chowder

- **CEREALS:** Oats are a standby low GL staple, but mix it up; you could experiment with bulgar, couscous or quinoa – it's high in protein and fibre, easy to cook and a good source of iron

- **DAIRY:** Milk products, though full of protein and calcium, can also be high in fat. Opt for low-fat

alternatives – and save the cheese board for tomorrow.
Fat-free or low-fat yoghurt will bring protein,
potassium (and, if you want them, pro-biotics) along
to the party, and, like nuts, it will help you feel fuller
longer. But beware; it can also be high in sugar.

Whatever you eat on a fast day (or any day), the most important thing is to relish it. Go slow. Have a look at the menu plans on pages 139-61 for more ideas.

I know I need plenty of veg, but should I eat it raw or cooked?

There is some debate as to whether vegetables are best eaten raw or cooked; cooking may, as raw-foodists contend, destroy vitamins, minerals and enzymes, but it also softens cellulose fibres, making nutrients more available for take-up in the body. Lycopene, a potent antioxidant found in tomatoes, is boosted in cooking.[37] A small blob of ketchup is no bad thing. Meanwhile, boiled or steamed carrots, spinach, mushrooms, asparagus, cabbage, peppers and many other vegetables also supply more antioxidants, such as carotenoids and ferulic acid, to the body than they do when raw.[38] The downside of cooking veg is that it can destroy their vitamin C. The raw versus cooked argument is a complicated one. Our best advice? Eat plenty of vegetables, just the way you like them.

Can I eat what I like on off-duty days?

Counter-intuitive as it may seem, no foods are off-limits, none proscribed. On the five days a week when we're not restricting calories, we both eat fish and chips, roast potatoes, biscuits, cake.

The whole point of the 5:2 approach is that for five days a week you shouldn't feel as if you are on a continuous, diet. Even so, don't try to gorge in a bid to make up for lost time, like a contestant in a blueberry pie contest. You could compensate for fasting by grossly overeating the next day, but it's very hard to do and you probably won't want to. We are creatures of habit, which makes it difficult for us to change our ways. But ingrained habits can also be helpful – after a fast people seem to find it relatively easy to step back into normal eating.

This absence of 'hyperphagia' (excessive appetite) after a day of rationing calories may seem surprising, but it is borne out by anecdotal experience. Many fasters report not feeling particularly hungry the day after a fast; what's more, many people discover that their life-long love of high-sugar, high-fat foods seems to diminish as Intermittent Fasting becomes a way of life. As yet, we can only speculate as to why this may be the case, but some individuals certainly experience a galvanizing effect from the weight loss they achieve: as they drop the pounds, their resolve grows stronger and eating more healthily, cutting back on pizzas, pies and potatoes, seems a natural lifestyle change.

Humans have, however, evolved to prefer calorie-rich foods – it once gave us an edge – and perhaps the greatest advantage of the Fast Diet is that it expressly includes 'pleasure foods', on five days of the week. For most of the time, there is no limitation, no deprivation, no guilt. The psychological impact of not being denied is huge; it frustrates what's known as the 'disinhibition effect' – a paradox in which designating certain foods 'off limits' makes us likely to eat more of them.[39]

Remember, then, that this is not a cycle of bingeing and starving: it is calibrated and moderate. Studies and experience show that Intermittent Fasting will regulate the appetite, not make it more extreme. You could pig out on your non-fast days, working your way steadily through all the ice-cream flavours in the freezer. (Even if you did, you'd still get some of the metabolic benefits of fasting.) But you won't do that. In all likelihood, you'll remain gently, intuitively attentive to your calorie intake, almost without noticing.

Similarly, you may find yourself naturally favouring healthier foods once your palate is modified by your occasional fasts. So, yes, eat freely, forbid nothing, but trust your body to say 'when'.

Is breakfast important?

Dieting lore has long suggested that breakfast is the most important meal of the day – miss it in the morning and it's like leaving the house without a coat. But that's not necessarily the case. Recent research shows that a bigger breakfast begets a bigger lunch (and a bigger dinner), which – no surprises here – means a higher overall calorie count for the day.[40] Some fasters find that they need sustenance to start the day, others may prefer to wait until later to 'break their fast'. It's up to you, and whichever pattern you choose may change over time.

What can I drink?

Plenty – as long as it doesn't have a substantial calorie content. In practice, as with most decisions on the Fast Diet, the choice is entirely up to you. Drink plenty of water – it's calorie-free, actually free, more filling than you think and will stop you confusing thirst for hunger. In summer, add rounds of cucumber or a dash of lime. Freeze it and suck on cubes. If you want warmth, miso soup contains protein, feels like food and clocks up only 84 calories per cup; vegetable bouillon pulls off the same trick. If you find it hard to sleep, a mug of instant low-cal hot chocolate is under 40 calories and a comforting thought.

During the day no-cal drinks are best. Hot water with lemon is a standby favourite for fasters, but you might prefer to add mint leaves or a scattering of cloves, a slice of ginger root or some lemongrass. If you are fond of herbal teas, try some unfamiliar flavours to spice up the day (liquorice and cinnamon, lemon grass and ginger, lavender, rose and chamomile...) Green tea may have health-giving antioxidant properties (the jury's out), but if you like it, drink it.

On fast days we drink our tea and coffee black and sugarless; if you prefer it with milk and artificial sweeteners, fine. But beware that the calories in milk add up, and what you are trying to do is extend the time you are not consuming any calories at all.

While fruit juices are seen as healthy, they generally have a surprisingly high sugar content, are lower in fibre than a whole fruit and can rack up the stealth calories without so much as a by-your-leave. Commercial smoothies can have a similar sugar content to Coke and, because they are acidic, they are corrosive to your teeth; they are also loaded with calories. If you need flavour, swap juice and smoothies for very dilute cordials – perhaps a dash of elderflower with fizzy water and lots of ice.

What about alcohol?

Alcoholic drinks, though pleasant, merely provide 'empty' calories. One glass of white wine contains about 120, while a 550ml can of beer has 250. Unless you really can't say no, abstain absolutely on a fast day – it's a golden opportunity to slash your weekly consumption without feeling serially deprived. Think of it as an alcovoid, for two achievable days each week.

And caffeine?

There's a growing body of evidence to suggest that – far

from being a guilty pleasure – drinking coffee may be good for you, helping to prevent mental decline, improve cardiac health and reduce the risk of liver cancer and stroke.[41] So go ahead, drink coffee if that's what gets you going and keeps you going each day. It's a useful weapon in your arsenal against boredom, and coffee breaks can pleasantly punctuate your day. There's no metabolic reason to avoid caffeine during a fast, but if you have trouble sleeping, limit your intake later in the day. You should, of course, drink it black. A 16 fl oz caramel macchiato has 224 calories… Just saying.

How about snacks?

The general idea of the Fast Diet is to give your body an occasional holiday from eating. Let your mouth rest. Give your belly a break. If you must snack on a fast day, do it with awareness and frugality, always keeping a weather eye on the GI:

	GI	GL
NUTS	27	3
POPCORN	72	8
RICE CAKES	80	19
FRUIT BARS	93	20
MARS BAR	65	26

You knew that chocolate bars were hardly a health food, but did you know how sugary rice cakes and fruit bars can be? Bear in mind that processed foods tend to have hidden sugars and, though convenient, won't give you anything like the nutritional advantage of good old-fashioned plants and proteins. Try carrot or celery sticks with hummus, or a handful of nuts – always factoring them into your daily calorie count (don't cheat).

Habitual snacking, even on low-calorie, nutrient-rich foods, is not advised; part of the motive here is to retrain your appetite, so don't overstimulate it. If your mouth is desperate for attention, give it a drink.

Can I use meal-replacement shakes to get me through the early days?

A number of people say that commercially available meal-replacement shakes helped them through the first, and normally hardest, weeks of an intermittent fast. Arguably, shakes are simpler than calorie-counting, and on your fast day you could simply sip away when waves of hunger strike. We are not great fans as we think real food is better. But if you find it helps, by all means try it. It's best to go for brands that are low in sugar.

What are the implications of cheating and having a few crisps or a cookie?

To clarify: this is a book about fasting, the voluntary abstention from eating food. The reasons why this is good for you go way beyond the fact that you are simply eating fewer calories. They arise because our bodies are designed for intermittent fasts. As you've seen, the scientific term is hormesis; what does not kill you makes you stronger. So while starvation is bad, a little bit of short, sharp, shock food restriction is good.

Your aim, then, is to carve out a food-free breathing space for your body. Going to 510 calories (or 615 for a man) won't hurt – it won't obliterate a fast. Indeed, the idea of slashing calories to a quarter of your daily intake on a fast day is simply one that has been clinically proven to have systemic effects on the metabolism. While there's no particular 'magic' to 500 or 600 calories, do try to stick resolutely to these numbers; you need clear parameters to make the strategy effective in the medium term.

Having 'an extra cookie' on a fast day would be antithetical to your goals (not to mention the fact that it would probably spike your blood sugar and eat up most of your allowance in one buttery bite); when you're fasting, you need to think sensibly and coherently about your food choices, following the plan laid out here. Exercise will-power, reminding yourself that tomorrow is on its way.

Should I take supplements during my fast?

The Fast Diet is an intermittent method, not a deprivation regime, so your nutritional intake from a wide variety of food sources should remain relatively steady over time, providing all the vitamins and minerals you require. If, as recommended, your fast-day foods centre on protein and plants, they'll give you all the goodness you need so you won't have to resort to costly bottled multivitamins. Do, however, choose your fast-day foods with care, ensuring that, over the course of a week, you consume adequate B vitamins, omega 3s, calcium and iron. Be sensible and eat well. While we are not fans of bottled vitamins and minerals, if a qualified health professional has suggested a particular supplement, you should continue to take it.

Should I exercise on a fast day?

Why not? In the interests of flexibility and normality, there's no reason to change your usual pattern of activity while fasting. Research demonstrates that even a more extreme three-day total fast has no negative effect on the ability to perform short-term, high-intensity workouts or long-duration, moderate-intensity exercise. Athletes seem to suffer no loss in performance during occasional fasting; a 2008 study of Tunisian footballers during Ramadan found that fasting had no effect on performance ('Each player was assessed for speed, power, agility, endurance, and for passing and dribbling skills. No variables were negatively affected by fasting.')[42]

In fact – and this is worth noting if you are aiming for optimal fitness – training while fasting can result in better metabolic adaptations[43] (which means enhanced performance over time), improved muscle protein synthesis,[44] and a higher anabolic response to post-exercise feeding.[45, 46]

Training on an empty stomach turns out to be beneficial on multiple levels, coaxing the body to burn a greater percentage of fat for fuel instead of relying on recently consumed carbs; if you're burning fat, don't forget: you're not storing it. As we've seen, one recent study found that working out before breakfast is beneficial for metabolic performance and weight loss.[47] A report in *The New York Times* suggests that it even 'blunts the deleterious effects of over-indulging' – making fasted exercise a canny way of 'combating Christmas'.[48] According to the study's authors, 'Our current data indicate that exercise training in the fasted state is more effective than exercise in the carbohydrate-fed state.' Certainly food for thought. Do not, however, increase your fast-day food allowance to 'compensate' for calories burned through exercise: on a fast day, stick to 500 or 600 calories, whatever level of activity you choose. That's where the benefits lie.

Are there gender differences in response to Intermittent Fasting ?

Clearly, men and women have metabolic and hormonal differences; for evolutionary reasons, we store and utilise fat in different ways. Women carry more fat, are better at storing it and tend to be more efficient at burning fat in response to exercise.[49] Though few studies have been done, there's some evidence to suggest that fasting women have a better response to endurance training than weight training,[50] while men may fare better with weights. Anecdotally, men tend to find working out on an empty stomach easier to accomplish than women.

In terms of general health, the benefits of occasional, short-term fasting for both sexes are pretty clear. Although quite a few studies have been done with male volunteers, others have been done with a mixed group or mainly female volunteers. The volunteers who took part in Michelle Harvie's studies, well over 200 of them, were all women. Their results are striking and positive; nevertheless, further trials are required to analyse the precise effects of fasting on hormones, particularly among women of different ages. As with all recommendations in this book, be cautious and self-aware. This is not meant to be a struggle; it's intended as a well-marked route to good health. If, for whatever reason, short bouts of fasting interrupt your cycle or your sleep pattern, modify your approach till you find a comfortable balance that works for you.

Can I fast if I'm trying to get pregnant?

The science is still unfolding, and there haven't been enough clinical trials to assess the overall effects of fasting on fertility. According to Professor Mark Mattson, an Intermittent Fasting plan, such as the Fast Diet, will not affect fertility. More extreme fasting may. It does in animals, but in a reversible manner. Nonetheless, we err on the side of caution and suggest that if you are trying to get pregnant, you should not fast. Period.

You should certainly not fast if you are already pregnant. Pregnant women should eat according to government guidelines and not limit their calorie intake.

Who else shouldn't fast?

There are certain groups for whom fasting is not advised. Type 1 diabetics are included in this list, along with anyone suffering from an eating disorder. If you are already extremely lean, do not fast. Children should never fast; they are still growing and should not be subject to nutritional stress of any type. If you have an underlying medical condition, visit your GP, as you would before embarking on any weight-loss regime.

Will I get headaches?

If you do, it may be due to dehydration rather than a lack of calories. You might experience mild withdrawal symptoms from sugar (or caffeine if you've dropped it), but the brevity of your fast shouldn't make this of particular concern. Keep drinking water. Treat a headache as you would normally; if fasting today is making you feel particularly unwell, stop. You are in charge.

Should I worry about low blood sugar?

If in reasonable good health, your body is a remarkably efficient and functional machine, capable of – in fact, designed for – the effective regulation of blood sugar. Short-term fasting is unlikely to yield a hypoglycaemic response. The recently propagated idea that we need to graze to avoid a 'blood sugar crash' is a myth; if you follow the guidelines set out here and eat low-GI foods on a fast day, your blood glucose should remain stable. But don't overdo it. If you fast for extended periods, longer than the bi-weekly, 24-hour modified eating programme recommended here, you may experience a drop in blood pressure, a drop in glucose levels and dizziness. So, fast smart. If you are diabetic, consult your doctor before embarking on any dietary change.

Will I feel tired?

Short-term, deliberate, modified fasting will not leave you beat – some fasters even report an energy boost on a Fast Day and beyond. As in normal life, you'll undoubtedly have up days and down days, good days and bad. Anecdotally, many Intermittent Fasters we have encountered report an increase in energy rather than a depletion. See how you fare. You may find that a fast day ends earlier than usual – no alcohol and plentiful sleep being a great way to arrive at breakfast sooner.

But will I go to bed hungry?

Probably not, though it will depend on your particular metabolism, and how you timed your fast-day calorie consumption. If you feel hungry, take your mind off it – a bubble bath, a good book, a stretch out, a herbal tea. Get psychology on your side: congratulate yourself on reaching the end of another fast day. Surprisiingly, perhaps, fasters report that they don't wake up ravenous and run to the fridge as soon as the alarm goes off. Hunger is a subtle beast, and your appetite will soon find its rhythm.

Will my body go into 'starvation mode' and hang on to fat?

Since you're not restricting calories every day, your body will not enter the fabled 'starvation mode'. Your fasting will never be intense. It will only ever be conservative and short-lived, so while your body will burn energy from its fat stores, it will not consume muscle tissue. Research has shown that occasional fasting does not suppress the metabolism.[51] Even extreme fasting – an absolute fast for three consecutive days[52] or on every other day for three weeks[53] – generates no decrease in basal metabolic rate. Nor does Intermittent Fasting raise levels of the hunger-stimulating hormone ghrelin. Researchers at Pennington Biomedical Research Center in Louisiana found that 'ghrelin was unchanged in both the men and the women, even after 36 hours of fasting'.[54] If you follow the moderate, judicious approach advised here, a short window without food is a scientifically sanctioned path to health and wellbeing.

What if everyone around me is eating on one of my fast days?

Participate, but with a nonchalant awareness. While support from family and friends is an asset, making a song and dance about your fast will only cause you to feel self-conscious, turning the diet into an obstruction, a hurdle, rather than something that should slot happily and calmly into your life. Remember your trump card: you'll eat normally again tomorrow. Some days, of course, are tougher than others. Naturally enough, you may find yourself feeling hungrier and less able to fast successfully when celebrating or attending events that revolve around food.

If you know that you have a social event in the diary, fast the day before or the day after. The flexibility of the plan explicitly means – in fact, it demands – that you still go to that wedding, birthday, anniversary dinner, christening, bar mitzvah, supper date, posh restaurant. Take a break for Christmas, Easter, Thanksgiving, Diwali. Yes, you may well put on a little weight, but this is a life, not a life sentence. You can always deviate, eat chips and dips and things on sticks, and then revert to more challenging fasting once the party's over.

What if I'm currently obese?

Clinical trials have concluded that Intermittent Fasting is a sustainable – indeed, one of the most effective – ways for obese individuals to lose weight and keep it off; the larger you are, the greater your initial weight loss is likely to be. If you are obese it's likely that, for whatever reason, traditional restrictive diets have failed for you. The Fast Diet is different because of its flexibility, its war on guilt, and its express approval of 'pleasure foods' on non-fast days. Studies done by Dr Michelle Harvie and Professor Tony Howell, cited above, have shown that most overweight women are able to adapt to calorie restricting two days a week and lose significant amounts of fat, even those who have had long-term weight issues. As with any underlying medical condition, we recommend that you fast under supervision.

Should I add a third day if I want to see accelerated results?

As Michael wrote earlier in this book, there is good scientific evidence from trials run by Dr Krista Varady and her team at the University of Illinois in Chicago of benefits from more rigorous Intermittent Fasting. They have done a number of carefully controlled studies where volunteers have tried Alternate Day Fasting (ADF). This form of Intermittent Fasting entails cutting calories every other day – a 500 calorie allowance for women, 600 for men. Most volunteers who took part in these studies lost significant amounts of weight, mainly as fat, and saw marked improvements in their biomarkers, including cholesterol.

I'm already slim enough, but would like to enjoy the health benefits of Intermittent Fasting. Is that possible?

If you are already at a reasonable, happy weight, you can still fast effectively, but consider adapting your consumption on non-fast days to encompass more calorie-dense foods. The main researchers we talked to in

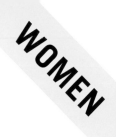

FAST 500 MENU PLANS

Breakfast: Porridge and blueberries
Dinner: Chicken stir-fry
Calories: *494*

Breakfast: Cottage cheese with pear and fig
Dinner: Sashimi and a tangerine
Calories: *483*

Breakfast: Yoghurt, blueberries and ham
Dinner: Feta Nicoise
Calories: *490*

Breakfast: Boiled egg & grapefruit
Dinner: Vegetarian Chilli
Calories: *500*

Breakfast: Smoked salmon, cracker and light cream cheese
Dinner: Thai salad
Calories: *497*

Breakfast: Scrambled eggs and smoked salmon
Dinner: Roasted vegetable salad. Tangerines
Calories: *494*

Breakfast: Boiled egg, ham and tangerine
Dinner: Mexican Pizza
Calories: *498*

FAST 600 MENU PLANS

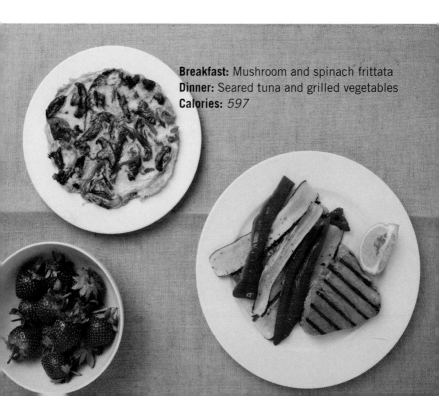

Breakfast: Mushroom and spinach frittata
Dinner: Seared tuna and grilled vegetables
Calories: *597*

Breakfast: Boiled eggs, asparagus, toast and plums
Dinner: Thai steak salad
Calories: *588*

Breakfast: Bacon, sausage, mushroom and spinach
Dinner: Roast mackerel and broccoli
Calories: *592*

Breakfast: Yoghurt with chopped banana, strawberries, blueberries and almonds
Dinner: Prawn, watercress and avocado salad. Tangerine
Calories: *591*

Breakfast: Smoked salmon
Dinner: Roast pork with cauliflower and broccoli
Calories: *580*

Breakfast: Simple muesli with grated apple
Dinner: No-carb caesar salad
Calories: *593*

Breakfast: Poached eggs on toast and raspberries
Dinner: Roast salmon with tomatoes and beans
Calories: *592*

this field are all slim and they still fast. With practice, you will discover an amicable balance between fasting and feeding which keeps your weight in the prescribed range. Fast once a week, rather than twice a week. There have been no specific studies to illuminate the effects of doing this, but use your common sense and watch the scales; don't slide. As mentioned above, if you are already extremely lean or suffering from an eating disorder, fasting of any description is not advised. If in doubt, see your GP.

Is it too late to start?
On the contrary, there's no time to lose. The Fast Diet is likely to prolong your life. It will moderate your appetite and help you lose weight. Its effects are quickly felt, often within a week of starting your simple bi-weekly mini fasts. It all points to a healthier, leaner, longer old age, fewer doctors' appointments, more energy, greater resistance to disease. Our advice? Start yesterday.

How long should I continue?
Interestingly, the Fast Diet's on/off eating scheme looks a lot like the approach of many naturally slim people. Some days they'll pick, other days they'll tuck into treats. In the long run, this is how the Fast Diet goes. As you settle into the routine, you'll naturally moderate your calorie intake on fast days and feed days, until the process is innate. When you reach your target weight, you can change the

frequency of your fast. Play with it. But don't drift; stay alert. Your aim is a permanent life change, not a blip, not a fad, not a dinner-party chat. This is a long-distance route to sustained weight loss. Accept that it is something you will do, in a form that suits you, indefinitely. For as long as life.

The future of fasting: where next?

Fasting, as we mentioned at the beginning of the book, has been practised for many thousands of years and yet science is only just starting to catch up. The first evidence of the long-term benefits of calorie restriction were found just over 80 years ago, when nutritionists working with rats at Cornell University in the US discovered that if you severely restrict the amount they eat, they live longer. Much longer.

Since then, the evidence has continued to mount that animals not only live longer, healthier lives if they are calorie-restricted, they also do so if they are intermittently starved. In recent years the research has moved on from rodents to humans and we are seeing the same patterns of improvement.

So where do we go from here? Professor Valter Longo, who has done so much pioneering work with IGF-1, is running a number of human trials in conjunction with colleagues at the University of Southern California, looking at the impact of fasting on cancer. They have already demonstrated that fasting will cut your risk of developing cancer; now they want to see if fasting will also improve the efficacy of chemotherapy and radiotherapy.

Dr Michelle Harvie and Professor Tony Howell, who work at the Genesis Breast Cancer Prevention Centre in Manchester, have done a great deal of fascinating work developing and testing different forms of two-day intermittent energy restriction. In this book we have quoted a couple of their studies – involving hundreds of female volunteers – which have shown that people can lose weight just as effectively by calorie restricting on an intermittent basis as by calorie restricting every day.

They are planning further studies, comparing what they call 'The 2-Day Diet' with standard dieting. These studies will undoubtedly add to our understanding of how well people are able to tolerate different patterns of eating in the long run.

Professor Mark Mattson of the National Institute on Aging in Baltimore is adding all the time to the dozens of research papers he has already published on the effects of fasting and Intermittent Fasting on the brain. We are particularly interested to see the outcome of some of his current studies, which include looking further into what happens to the brains of volunteers when put on an Intermittent Fasting regime.

In addition, his team is looking at drug therapies, as they know that despite the benefits, many people may not want to fast. So they are, for example, investigating a drug called Byetta, used for the treatment of diabetes, but which also seems to activate the production of BDNF (brain-derived neurotrophic factor). This in turn, as we've seen, seems to protect the brain against the ravages of ageing. The hope is that Byetta or a related drug will, if not prevent dementia, at least slow its progression significantly.

Intermittent Fasting has, until now, been one of the best-kept secrets in science. We look forward, with a great deal of personal interest, to seeing how this particular story unfolds.

THE FAST DIET EATING PLAN

FAST-DAY COOKING TIPS

1. Feel free to bump up the quantities of leafy, low-calorie, low-GI vegetables given here. It is difficult to pig out on leafy veg, and if you need bulk, here's where you should get it. Roasted veg are tasty. Lightly steamed is best. Invest in a tiered bamboo steamer, and cook your proteins and veggies in several health-packed, eco-friendly levels.

2. Some vegetables benefit from cooking, others are better eaten raw. See page 113 for more details. Cooking certain veg – including carrots, spinach, mushrooms, asparagus, cabbage and peppers – breaks down the cell structure without destroying vitamins, allowing you to absorb more goodies. For raw vegetables, a mandolin makes preparation easy and swift.

3. Fast days should be low fat, rather than no fat. A teaspoon of olive oil can be used in cooking or drizzled over vegetables for flavour; or use a cooking-oil spray to get a thin film. Nuts and fattier meats such as pork are included in the plans. Do include a light oil dressing on your salads; it means that you are more likely to absorb their fat-soluble vitamins.

4. The acid in lemon or orange dressings means that you will absorb more iron from leafy greens such as spinach and kale. Watercress with orange is a great combination, perhaps scattered with some sesame and sunflower seeds or blanched almonds, for a little protein and crunch.

5. Always cook with a non-stick pan to cut down on calorie-dense fats. Add a splash of water if the food sticks.

6. Weigh your food after preparing it, so that the calorie count is correct.

7. Dairy is also included here: choose lower-fat cheeses and semi-skimmed milk, avoiding full-fat yoghurts in favour of low-fat alternatives. Drop the lattes and bin the butter on a fast day: they are calorie traps.

8. Similarly, avoid starchy white carbohydrates (bread, potatoes, pasta) and opt instead for low-GI carbs such as vegetables, pulses and slow-burn cereals. Choose brown rice and quinoa. Porridge for breakfast will keep you fuller for longer than a commercial cereal.

9. Ensure that you get some fibre in your fast: eat the skin of apples and pears, have oats for breakfast, keep those leafy vegetables coming in.

10. Add flavour where you can: chilli flakes will give a kick to any savoury dish. Vinegars, including balsamic, will lend acidity. Add fresh herbs too – they are virtually calorie-free, but give personality to a plate.

11. Eating protein will help keep you fuller longer. Stick to the low-fat proteins, including some nuts and legumes. Remove the skin and fat from meat before cooking.

12. Soup can be a saviour on a hungry day, particularly if you choose a light broth packed with leafy veg (a Vietnamese pho would be ideal, though hold back on the noodles). Soup is satiating, and a good way of using up ingredients languishing in the fridge.

13. Use agave as a sweetener if required; it's low-GI.

FAST 500 MENU PLANS FOR WOMEN

Breakfast *142 calories*
Half a tub of cottage cheese (100g, 78 calories)
One sliced pear (100g, 40 calories)
One fresh fig (55g, 24 calories)

Dinner *341 calories*
<u>Sashimi:</u> 3-5 pieces salmon (100g, 180 calories) and tuna (100g, 136 calories) – served with soy sauce, wasabi and ginger

1 tangerine (70g, 25 calories)

Daily total: 483

DAY 2

Breakfast *197 calories*
Porridge made with 40g oats (160 calories) and water. Top with 75g of blueberries (37 calories)

Dinner *306 calories*
Chicken stir-fry: cut chicken fillet cut into strips (140g oz, 148 calories). Fry in a non-stick pan in a tsp olive oil (27 calories) with a tsp finely chopped ginger (2 calories), a tbsp chopped coriander (3 calories), clove of crushed garlic (3 calories), 2 tsp soy sauce (3 calories) and half a squeezed lemon (1 calorie) until browned and sealed, adding water if chicken sticks. Add a handful sugar snap peas (50g, 12 calories), 100g finely sliced cabbage (26 calories) and 2 carrots cut into thin strips (160g, 56 calories), and cook for 5-10 more minutes until the chicken is cooked, adding water if necessary

1 tangerine (70g/2.5 oz, 25 calories)

Daily total: 503

DAY 3

Breakfast *125 calories*
1 boiled egg (61g, 90 calories)
Half a grapefruit (115g, 35 calories)

Dinner *378 calories*
<u>Vegetarian chilli</u>: fry a clove of garlic (3 calories) and half a
finely chopped red chilli in a tsp olive oil (27 calories).
Add a pinch of cumin and 1 large or 4 small chopped
mushrooms (20g, 3 calories) and cook for five minutes,
adding water if it sticks. Add half a tin of chopped tomatoes
(200g, 32 calories) and half a tin of kidney beans (200g,
200 calories), stir and simmer for 10 mins. Serve with 2 tbsp
cooked wild brown rice (80g, 113 calories)

Daily total: 503

DAY 4

Breakfast *194 calories*
Smoked salmon (112g, 159 calories)
1 plain Ryvita (35 calories) spread with a tsp light cream cheese (11 calories)

Dinner *303 calories*
Thai salad: put 2 tbsp of Thai fish sauce (20 calories), the juice of one lime (20g, 1 calorie), a tsp sugar (16 calories), 2 sliced spring onions (20g, 5 calories) and 1 red chilli, finely chopped (1 calorie) into a bowl. Mix well. Add 10 small cooked prawns (30g, 30 calories) 2 grated carrots (160g, 56 calories) and 50g vermicelli noodles (194 calories), soaked according to instructions. Toss well

Daily total: 497 calories

DAY 5

Breakfast *171 calories*
<u>Strawberry smoothie:</u> blend a banana (100g, 95 calories),
a pot of fat-free natural yoghurt (150g, 62 calories), a large
handful of strawberries (50g, 14 calories), a splash of
water and some ice until thick and creamy.
Serve immediately

Dinner *325 calories*
<u>Oven-baked smoked haddock:</u> place a fillet of smoked
haddock (200g, 202 calories) on a non-stick baking tray
and roast for 15–20 minutes, until fish is cooked through.
Serve with a poached egg (61g, 90 calories) and sprigs of
lightly steamed tender stem broccoli (100g, 33 calories)

Daily total: 496 calories

DAY 6

Breakfast *233 calories*
<u>Dipped apple:</u> slice one apple (100g, 47 calories) and one mango (150g, 86 calories) and serve with 2 tbsp of half-fat crème fraîche 'dip' (100 calories)

Dinner *255 calories*
<u>Tuna, bean and garlic salad:</u> put 140g canned cannellini beans (108 calories), 120g good-quality canned tuna in spring water (119 calories), 6 chopped cherry tomatoes (90g, 16 calories) and a generous handful of baby leaf spinach (30g, 8 calories) in a salad bowl. Mix well. Drizzle over a dressing made from 1 clove of crushed garlic (3 calories), the juice and zest of 1 lemon (1 calorie) and a splash of white wine vinegar

Daily total – 488 calories

DAY 7

Breakfast *140 calories*
1 boiled egg (90 calories)
A slice of ham (23g, 25 calories)
One tangerine (25 calories)

Dinner *358 calories*
Mexican pizza: take 1 tortilla (55g, 144 calories) and top
with 2 tbsp passata (5 calories), 3 small diced balls of light
mozzarella (90g, 159 calories), and scatter with chopped
vegetables: mushrooms, red pepper, courgette, red onion,
aubergine, spinach are all OK (170g, 50 calories). Cook in hot
oven for 5-10 minutes

Daily total – 498 calories

DAY 8

Breakfast *256 calories*
<u>Scrambled eggs:</u> add a splash of skimmed milk (15g, 5 calories) to 2 beaten eggs (180 calories) and scramble in a non-stick frying pan (no added oil or butter). Chop 50g smoked salmon (71 calories) and stir into the eggs

Dinner *238 calories*
<u>Roasted vegetable salad:</u> mix together 10 cherry tomatoes (150g, 27 calories), with half a sliced courgette (50g, 9 calories), half a sliced aubergine (75g, 11 calories), 1 sliced red pepper (160g, 51 calories). Scatter with basil leaves (1 calorie) and drizzle with balsamic vinegar. Roast in a hot oven for 20—25 minutes. Serve with 2 tbsp Parmesan (20g, 90 calories)

2 tangerines (140g, 50 calories)

Daily total – 494 calories

DAY 9

Breakfast *140 calories*
1 small pot of natural fat-free yoghurt (150g, 62 calories)
50g blueberries (28 calories)
Two slices ham (46g, 50 calories)

Dinner *360 calories*
Feta Niçoise: chop and mix together 1 egg (90 calories), a
handful of lettuce (20g, 3 calories), a handful of cooked green
beans (50g, 12 calories), and 100g chopped cucumber (10
calories). Top with 90g crumbled feta cheese (225 calories),
six black olives (18g, 19 calories) and 1 tbsp chopped parsley
(1 calorie). Drizzle with white wine vinegar to serve

Daily total – 500 calories

Breakfast *280 calories*
100g grilled kipper (280 calories)

Dinner *217 calories*
Fast-day Insalata Caprese: slice 3 small balls of low-fat
mozzarella (90g, 159 calories) and place on a plate with 1
sliced beef tomato (150g, 27 calories). Scatter with fresh
basil and drizzle with good-quality balsamic vinegar (3ml, 6
calories)

8 strawberries (96g, 26 calories)

Daily total – 497

FAST 600 MENU PLANS FOR MEN

DAY 1

Breakfast *271 calories*
Mushroom and spinach frittata: fry half a sliced onion (75g, 27 calories) in 1 tsp of olive oil (27 calories). Add 4 small chopped mushrooms (20g, 3 calories). Cook until tender. Add a generous handful of spinach (30g, 8 calories); cook for 2 minutes. Pour over 2 beaten eggs (180 calories). Cook for 5 minutes, and finish under a hot grill until eggs are set

12 strawberries (96g, 26 calories)

Dinner *326 calories*
Seared tuna: heat a griddle pan and sear a tuna steak (168g, 229 calories) on both sides using no fat, but squeezing in lemon if necessary. Serve with 1 whole grilled small red pepper (120g, 52 calories) and 1 sliced, grilled courgette (100g, 18 calories). Cut the pepper and courgette into long strips (for the courgette, about $1/2$cm wide). Mix in a bowl with 1 tsp olive oil (27 calories), season, and grill on medium-high heat for 5 minutes each side. Dress with a squeeze of lemon

Daily total – 597 calories

DAY 2

Breakfast *288 calories*
2 poached eggs (180 calories) on a slice of wholemeal toast
(31g, 78 calories)
30 raspberries (120g, 30 calories)

Dinner *304 calories*
Roast salmon: place a 140g salmon fillet (252 calories) with
10 cherry tomatoes (150g, 27 calories) on the vine on a
baking tray. Bake at 200ºc for about 15–20 minutes until the
fish is cooked. Serve with a generous 112g helping of green
beans (25 calories)

Daily total – 592 calories

DAY 3

Breakfast *298 calories*
Simple muesli: Mix 50g oats (201 calories) with a grated apple (100g, 47 calories). Cover with skimmed milk (150ml, 50 calories)

Dinner *295 calories*
No-carb caesar salad: grill 2 slices of parma ham (34g, 76 calories) for 4-5 minutes, turning once, until crispy.
Slice 1 chicken breast (140g, 148 calories) into two. Grill for about 3–4 minutes each side or until cooked. Cut into pieces and place on a substantial bed of 100g chopped cos lettuce (16 calories). Serve with 1 tbsp grated Parmesan (45 calories), and 1 tbsp reduced-calorie Caesar salad dressing (15g, 10 calories –eg Sainsbury's Be Good To Yourself). Crumble the grilled Parma ham over the top

Daily total – 593 calories

DAY 4

Breakfast *330 calories*
100g grilled kipper (280 calories)
2 tangerines (50 calories)

Dinner *264 calories*
Marinated steak and Asian cabbage salad: Marinate a
piece of sirloin steak (90g, 120 calories) in a mixture of soy,
the juice of 1 lime and crushed garlic. Grill until cooked,
turning once. Serve with Asian cabbage salad: combine 1
grated carrot (80g, 28 calories) with 90g Savoy cabbage
(24 calories) cut into thin strips, and a handful of coriander
(1 calorie). *For dressing*, mix 1 tsp sugar (16 calories) with
1 tbsp Thai fish sauce (10 calories), the juice of 1 lime (2
calories), a crushed clove garlic (3 calories). Pour over salad
and top with 10g chopped roasted, unsalted peanuts (60
calories)

Daily total – 594 calories

DAY 5

Breakfast *177 calories*
2 lean grilled rashers of bacon (50g, 107 calories)
1 small sausage (20g, 59 calories)
1 small grilled portobello mushroom (20g, 3 calories)
A generous handful of spinach (30g, 8 calories)

Dinner *415 calories*
<u>Roast mackerel and vegetables:</u> place a mackerel fillet
(147g, 351 calories) on top of 2 sliced tomatoes (170g,
30 calories). Wrap in foil and roast in a hot oven for 10–15
minutes or until fish is done. Serve with a big pile of
tenderstem broccoli (100g, 33 calories) dressed with the juice
of half a lemon (1 calorie) and salt

Daily total – 592 calories

DAY 6

Breakfast *271 calories*
Small pot of natural fat-free yoghurt (150g, 62 calories)
1 chopped banana (100g, 95 calories)
Six strawberries (72g, 20 calories)
100g blueberries (100g, 25 calories)
Four almonds, chopped (8g, 69 calories)

Dinner *320 calories*
Prawn, watercress and avocado salad: mix 28g watercress
(6 calories) with 140g cooked prawns (139 calories), half
an avocado (72g, 137 calories), half a red onion (30g, 11
calories) chopped and 1 tbsp capers (2 calories). Dress with
white wine vinegar

1 tangerine (25 calories)

Daily total – 591 calories

Breakfast *261 calories*
Scrambled eggs: add a splash of skimmed milk (15ml, 5 calories) to 2 beaten eggs (180 calories) and scramble in a non-stick pan. Serve with one very small piece of Parma ham (34g, 76 calories)

Dinner *326 calories*
Spiced dhal: in 1 tsp olive oil (27 calories), fry a finely chopped small onion (60g, 22 calories), a clove of crushed garlic (3 calories) and 1 tsp finely chopped ginger (3 calories). Cook for 5 minutes. Add half a pint of water, 50g dried, washed red lentils (159 calories), a pinch of cumin, coriander, turmeric, cayenne pepper, salt and pepper. Boil for 20 mins or until lentils are tender. Garnish with 2 tbsn of fat-free natural yogurt (40 calories). Serve with 2 poppadoms (72 calories)

Daily total – 587 calories

DAY 8

Breakfast *331 calories*
2 boiled eggs (180 calories)
5 asparagus spears (125g, 33 calories), to dip
1 slice wholemeal toast (31g, 78 calories)
2 plums (110g, 40 calories)

Dinner *256 calories*
Thai steak salad: grill a sirloin steak (140g, 188 calories)
on both sides until cooked, and slice very thin. Serve on a
big pile of shredded lettuce (100g, 14 calories), and 100g
shredded Savoy cabbage (24 calories). Serve with this
dressing: juice of 1 lime (1 calorie), 1 tsp sugar (16 calories),
a crushed clove of garlic (3 calories), a chopped, deseeded
chilli (1 calorie) and 1 tbsp Thai fish sauce (10 calories)

Daily total – 588 calories

DAY 9

Breakfast *214 calories*
Smoked salmon (150g, 213 calories)
Lemon wedges to serve (1 calorie)

Dinner *383 calories*
<u>Roast pork:</u> serve 150g lean roast pork (289 calories) with
cauliflower (50g, 17 calories) and broccoli (50g, 17 calories).
Drizzle with 1 tbsp meat juices (60 calories)

Daily total – 597 calories

DAY 10

Breakfast *206 calories*
1 small 150g pot of fat-free, natural yoghurt (62 calories)
1 chopped banana (100g, 96 calories)
1 tbsp sugar-free muesli, not granola, stirred through (15g, 48 calories)

Dinner *386 calories*
Bacon & butterbean soup: fry two rashers of bacon (54g, 116 calories) in 1 tsp olive oil (27 calories) for 2 minutes. Add half a small finely chopped onion (30g, 11 calories), half a chopped leek (50g, 11 calories), half a finely sliced carrot (40g, 14 calories), and 1 diced stalk of celery (1 calorie). Cook for 5 minutes, adding a splash of water if it sticks. Add half a can of butterbeans (200g, 206 calories) and half a pint of water (250ml) and simmer for 20 minutes. Season. Blend until desired consistency, or simply mash for chunkier texture

Daily total – 592 calories

Menu plans by Sarah Maber

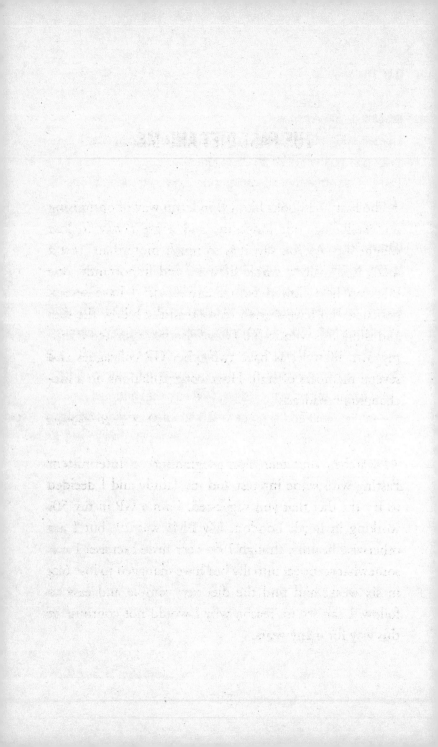

THE FAST DIET AND ME

❛ The Fast Diet looks like a wonderful way of optimising our wellbeing, our longevity, and a great way to lose weight too. As you say, it is so much more than "just a diet", it is really a whole lifestyle, and importantly, one that can be followed with relative ease. I have several patients who have started to successfully follow the diet and think it is wonderful. I have also incorporated it into my own lifestyle, as have two other GP colleagues and several members of staff. Huge congratulations on a life-changing broadcast.❜

Dr Pete Bridgwood

❛ I watched your television programme on Intermittent Fasting with some interest and my family and I decided to try the diet that you suggested. I am a GP in my 50s working in north London. My BMI was 29, but I am otherwise healthy, though I do very little exercise. I was somewhat sceptical initially but have managed to lose 6kg in six weeks and find the diet very simple and easy to follow. I can see no reason why I would not continue in this way for many years.

I have presented a summary of your programme to a few colleagues and have started to recommend it to some of my patients with startling results.

One particular patient, who obviously has metabolic syndrome and a family history of type 2 diabetes, had a fasting glucose of 7.2. After only a few weeks, his fasting glucose dropped to 5.9 and he lost 5kg in weight.

I would like to spread the word even further and wondered if you had plans to design a simple leaflet or website that I could either give to my patients or direct them to view on the Internet. I have difficulty explaining the diet in the short time at the end of one of my ten-minute consultations. I think that this type of manageable eating plan is likely to be so much more successful in managing the obesity epidemic than the current plans to "traffic light" and give fat and sugar contents on food packaging. I think it would be so much more useful to emphasise the calorie content of foods.'

Dr Jon Brewerton

'I have been on IF now for the last 14 weeks. I have lost 9.4lb and 9.5 inches. On previous diets I have never got below 140lb (ten stone).

Start weight	145.6lb
Current weight	136.4lb
Height	5'6"

Inch loss:

Bust	1.25"
Midriff	0.5"
Waist	1.75"
Abdomen	2.5"
Hips	2.5"
Thighs	0.5" from each leg

Improvements other than weight loss: eyes look brighter and clearer. More energy. Sleeping better. Clearer head and better mental clarity (although not tested, I feel that I can remember things more easily). Feel healthy.'

Sarah H

'A busy mum with three children, I was finding losing weight after having my youngest child really difficult. It didn't help being constantly surrounded by food and snacks, preparing three, sometimes four, meals a day for the family. I enjoy food and socialising, so restrictive diets just felt like a chore and a battle of will-power every day, so it was never long before I was back to square one.

The Fast Diet, for me, is a more manageable way to lose weight both physically and emotionally, as it's only two days a week of "being good" and sticking to 500 calories. It also fits beautifully around my social life, as the fast days can be flexible, so I make sure it's a feast day when I'm out for drinks or meals.

It's also not actually that hard to resist temptation for

one day, as I know that the next day I can have a donut or a curry and a few glasses of wine if I really want; and when I do, I enjoy it even more without feeling guilty.

The proof is, literally, in the pudding; I have been eating and enjoying them on feast days, but sticking to 500 calories on fast days, and I am still losing weight. This works.'

Clare Wilson

'Yesterday I ate really well as, although I can eat what I like, I'm also thinking that I don't want to undo all my hard work. So I did have a bag of crisps, and I did have pork and apple sausages in cider for tea with one of my daughter's homemade lemon pies afterwards, but I didn't have the ton of crap I normally have in between.

I don't think I find the fast days too hard because of the relatively short tunnel and there being light at the end of it. Looking forward to a weekend of eating normally though!

I think part of what this plan is getting at is that we need to learn it's OK to feel hungry, and in fact it is an essential part of being slim. I speak as a lifelong overeater – the FULL feeling is so normal for me and I had some weird fear about feeling hungry.

Well, guess what? It's not the end of the world. I live in a city with stores everywhere – I can have food at any moment I want, so hunger isn't a sign I'm about to perish or get weak.

During the last couple of months, I've been learning to

embrace feeling hungry and being comfortable with that – it's a sign from my body to eat again soon (and hopefully that it is burning fat now), not a sign to be feared.

It's OK to feel hungry. Immediate death from starvation will not occur.'

Unhappyhildebrand on Mumsnet.com

'Everyone is doing so well. You can really do anything for a day, and with a bit of planning I managed to plug most of my hunger pangs down to a manageable level. Scales were showing a good loss this morning.

Any concerns I had on my exercise performance while fasting were scuppered this morning. I ran my fastest sustained pace ever and that was following a 500-calorie fast day with no breakfast, only a coffee – I smell fat burning!!!! I feel great and will break the fast properly with lunch today. Next fast day is on Thursday. Good luck to everyone fasting today.'

SpringGoddess on Mumsnet.com

'Just wanted to add that exercising whilst fasting was fine for me, too. I spent an hour at the gym last night and felt good. Did 35 minutes on the cross trainer and some weights and didn't feel faint or dizzy. It's amazing how good I feel when fasting actually.'

dontcallmehon on Mumsnet.com

'I did Day One yesterday and am feeling brilliant this

morning and full of energy. In the end, I just decided to go as long as I could without food. I drank tea with milk and black coffee and water throughout the day. I had some melon and strawberries at 4pm, then a full dinner of two Quorn sausages, one boiled egg, one slice of toast, rocket salad with a bit of balsamic. It tasted so good! But, the fasting was easier than expected. Wasn't too hungry and just tried to keep busy during the day.'

Mondayschild78 on Mumsnet.com

'My Day One yesterday also went brilliantly! I wasn't even ravenous when I woke up this morning, I was able to wait an hour before having some Burgen bread toast and peanut butter – and I struggled to finish it! I loved the feeling of emptiness in my tummy, and the hunger pangs were also enjoyable at times – is this weird? My whole life I had eaten when I wasn't hungry because I was so scared of having a single tummy rumble. I am weirdly looking forward to my next fast day...'

ILoveStripeySocks on Mumsnet.com

'For me, fasting - 600 calories twice a week - has changed my attitude to food and drink. It has broken a cycle of over indulgence which caused my weight to rise steadily for 30 years. We are creatures of habit, and without realizing it slip into patterns of behavior which are difficult to change. But now something profound has happened: I perceive things more clearly and there is something about this new state of mind which reminds me of how I felt in my 20s when I had a BMI of around 22. I no longer feel comfortable if I have eaten too much, and I feel more in control. The habit is being broken. I suspect I will be on this diet more or less for the rest of my life.

David Cleevely

'I am now two weeks into my 5:2 diet and I am already seeing a positive effect on my weight. At my second weigh-in, I had lost a total of five pounds. Feel noticeably slimmer and happy that I can maintain this for a long time to come.

Stats	5' 10" male
Start weight	13st 9lb
Week 1	13st 6lb
Week 2	13st 4lb

Really enjoyed the programme!'

Nick Wilson

'OK, fast two of week 13 was completed yesterday and as promised, here's an update for a whole quarter of Intermittent Fasting.

The programme involves eating only 600 calories on two selected, non-consecutive days of the week. Apart from the two days a week, that's it. The rest of the time,

I eat and drink what I want. You don't need to exercise or count calories on a daily basis, you don't feel hungry 24/7 and, best of all, you don't die of starvation.

Tonight is Indian night, tomorrow is steak night and Sunday is probably Italian. Every night is booze night. That doesn't sound like too onerous a regime to me. It's fair to say that my overall weekly calorie consumption (excluding fast days) has reduced, not because I'm avoiding eating on the feed days, but purely because I'm just not as hungry.

Over the past 13 weeks, I've been developing the regime to suit myself and have got into a fairly settled Monday and Thursday routine. I consume nothing at all during the day apart from three or four teas/coffees (just marginally whitened) and about one to one and a half litres of tap water. I come home and I do a ten-mile thrash on a cycle turbo trainer. Last night, I did it in 30 minutes and 25 seconds, an average of 20mph for 30 minutes. Using that assumption, my ten-miler burns around 550 calories. By doing it before you eat on a fast day, the theory (I guess) is that you're forcing your body to burn body fat, rather than the carbs it would normally turn to for a short burst of energy.

Hunger wise – well, it's OK. I eat late prior to a fast day and that definitely helps. I find having even a small breakfast actually triggers hunger for the rest of the day, so I avoid everything until late on, when I have some flavoured rice (240 cals) and the rest as vegetables. It's easily managed – you actually don't get hungrier throughout the day and it's easy to take your mind off it by doing something. You DO have to approach a fast day in the right mindset though. If you don't, you'll have a pretty hellish time. Do it right and it's really quite a doddle.

So when I started the regime in mid-August, I was a fraction of a pound off 14 stone and on the last notch of my belt (I know that's not very scientific and I wish I'd taken more measurements when I started, but hey-ho).

This morning, I tipped the scales at 12st 9lbs and the fourth notch on my belt is quite comfortable (the third is a wee bit loose). One notch = just over one inch. The goal without exercise would be to lose a pound a week (given that a 4000 weekly calorie restriction = roughly 1 pound of body fat). With the one hour of exercise a week, I accelerated it by almost 50% to 19lbs in the same period.

I'm keeping going until Christmas where I hope to go to a 5:1+1 (the +1 being an 800 or 900 calorie day). If that works, then I'll stay on that for the rest of my time.

I went for a cycle last Sunday after having a full breakfast and it was incredibly easy. Loads of speed, the hills were actually fun and, apart from the chilliness, it was extremely enjoyable. The benefit of being fitter and having a fuelled-up body I guess. LOADS of energy.

Other benefits:

I have suffered from asthma since I was a child. It's

nowhere near as bad as it was when I was a bairn, but now it's practically disappeared. My "peak flow" reading has gone up by over 30 per cent in the 13 weeks – probably as a result of the weight loss allowing me to exercise harder.

A wee bit girly here, but I'd say my skin complexion has improved dramatically. No plooks or blackheads – even the touch of dry skin on my elbows has gone.'

David Norvell

❛Both my partner and I watched your programme and thought it was very interesting, so we decided to start 5:2 fasting on the following Monday. (Always good to start news things on a Monday, I find!) I have done liquid fasting in the past, for weeks, and really liked it. But then I put the weight back on again, I found. This seems to work better.

Height	1.60m
Weight	83kg

I'm not very FAT as such, but I do need to lose weight, especially around my tummy/waist – the exact place where it's not good for you to be fat... I know! My aim is to get to 65–70kg, but at my age, it's not as easy to lose weight as it used to be when I was younger (according to my GP).

6 Aug	83kg (started fasting)
8 Aug	82kg

9 Aug	81kg
14 Aug	81kg
18 Aug	80kg
23 Aug	80kg
27 Aug	79.5kg
6 Sept	79.5kg
13 Sept	78.5kg
21 Sept	79kg

We both love the Intermittent Fasting. As you can see, I have lost some weight and the only reason it has not gone quicker is the fact I have not done as much exercise as I set out to do originally. We will certainly continue and I will keep weighing myself to check the progress.

We also find it makes us want to eat less the adjacent days, too. We do our two days on Tuesdays and Wednesdays. Come Thursday morning, I feel so "light" and full of energy, I don't want to "spoil" it by eating too much even if it's my feeding day.

We have our main "fasting meal" in the evening, as it's the time we see each other at home after work, to settle down and talk over dinner. It's probably not ideal from a calorie-burning aspect, but it's more practical for us and suits us best.

A typical fasting day main meal:

- Corn on the cobs as starter.
- Salmon fillet with garlic, lemon, herbs, salt and

pepper and a minimum amount of olive oil OR a two-egg omelette with onion, garlic, parsley, sliced mushrooms.
• Salad: various green salad leaves, tomatoes, red onion, herbs, maybe beetroot.
• Drink: water

During the day, we eat a banana and an apple.

I'm really grateful for you making this programme and have passed it on to friends and family who have taken it on, too.'

Britt Warg

'I'm a neurophysiology and pharmacology student, researching Parkinson's. Inspired by your TV programme, I decided to "self-experiment". This has now blossomed into a project that will be run at my university. I'm interested in data, neurodegenerative disorders and what steps I can take in my own lifestyle that will decrease my occurrence of breast cancer. I am a two-time (and counting) breast cancer patient, so I'm rather interested in what impact (if any) Intermittent Fasting could have on recurrence.

From my blog, www.schrokit.wordpress.com:

It's Not a Diet
So seven weeks into 5:2 (or 2:5 as I like to call it since I think of my weeks starting with fasting and then five

days of EATING) and still going strong. I'm a little over a stone down, with Mr Schrokit not too far behind (he keeps calling his jeans "fat man trousers" since he needs to do up his belt a few extra notches inwards…)

Because the overall difference in my appearance and 'result' is so easy to see (though people keep asking me if I changed my hair, got new glasses etc., they can't seem to pin down the weight loss, but I'm getting compliments galore), when I talk to people about fasting, they seem VERY keen to give it a go. In fact, many of Mr Schrokit's colleagues are on this so-called "diet" and finding it very eye-opening about their own eating habits.

But it's not a diet. The best description I've heard so far is from blog commenter Gordon. It's a strategy, to quote him, and I can't think of a better word.

Aside from eating a healthy balanced diet, whatever all the trendy diet books tell you, weight control is really about the aggregate number of calories you consume in the long run. The thing that fasting does seem to do is to help one get back in touch with actual appetite. For example, hungry versus bored, or hungry v tired, hungry v craving and most of all, hungry versus thirsty all seem a bit more obvious after fasting a couple of days.'

Nicole Slavin

‘I've been doing the Intermittent Fasting diet for about

three months now and wrote a blog post about it.

As you see, my experiences have been positive. What I didn't mention on my blog is that my husband has high cholesterol, which is an inherited condition, and the main reason we went on this diet. He didn't need to lose more than a couple of kilos in weight (he's always been a racing snake), so now he makes sure he increases his calorie intake (healthily with homemade smoothies) during the five days.'

From my blog, www.helenahalme.blogspot.co.uk:

When I was younger and living in Helsinki I did a few complete fasting sessions with my father. This fast would last five days and we were only allowed to drink fruit juices on the first and last days. So I thought I knew what I was getting into.

But this diet, which basically means you eat less on two days per week, is much easier. You're allowed 500 calories (600 for men – so unfair!), which when you think about it isn't that bad. And unlike the fasts of my youth, on this one you're allowed to drink coffee. (Coffee is the one thing I cannot give up these days…)

I've been doing the fasting for about three months now, and have lost 5kgs. I feel so much better on it, not only because of the weight loss, but because I seem to have more energy and control over my eating… After the initial shock to the system, your stomach actually contracts and you feel less hungry, more aware of how much you eat on any given day, whether it is one of the two or one of the five days of the week.

So here are my five tips to successfully do this diet:

- Do not fast on consecutive days – it's too hard and I find the second day in a row gruelling. And don't do weekends – we tried a Friday and nearly killed each other.

- Get busy – the more you have to think about something else other than food, the easier it is. I work from home half of the week, so I try to fast when I'm in the office. And don't watch Nigella on TV while fasting. She's like a Domestic Devil to me on one of my two days.

- Get yourself an app. I use MyFitnessPal which is a simple tool to count calories. A notepad is equally good, but for those of you, like me, who love apps, this one also records the foods you've consumed, the exercise you take and the weight you are losing (and predicts what you would lose in five weeks if each day was like the one you've just recorded).

- Don't be too hard on yourself. I have missed a couple of fasting days during the past three months. Just because you do that, there's no need to throw in the towel. There's always tomorrow, or next week!

- Don't go alone. Doing this with someone is so much easier. Some weeks, because of schedules, my husband and I have had to do different days, and it just doesn't work.'

' We've been fasting since the beginning of September and it has worked for me in terms of weight loss and generally feeling healthier. I was 58.8kg and I'm now 50.9kg (note I'm 1.56m tall!). My partner has gone from 95kg to hovering around 87kg.

We find it is easy to stick to, with a bit of planning. Even during the Christmas season, I'm finding it much easier to manage than other eating plans. It seems like something we could stick to in the long term, even if we go down to once a week on some weeks. For now, twice a week works fine.

We end up splitting our calories into three meals. I'm vegetarian so we usually stick to soups and salads. In winter it is basically three meals of soup, or a banana or an egg for breakfast plus two soup meals. During warmer months, we had salad for lunch to mix it up.

I've converted quite a few people already. We all agree that we go to bed a little bit earlier and certainly looking forward to breakfast more than usual. Sometimes I vow to have the biggest, unhealthiest breakfast the next morning but always just end up having toast or cereal.

The main limitation I have found is exercise. I used to exercise most days and now I need to plan exercising around the fast days. I do Pilates or weights on fasting days, and stick to cardio on other days.'

Luella Charles

❛I watched your programme when it went out on TV in early August. It made good sense to me and I persuaded my husband to watch it too. Since then we have been following the fasting schedule (with 500 calories for me and 600 for him) most weeks, but not every week as sometimes we are only able to fit in a fast a week.

Our main motivation is for health benefits as we age (we are in our mid-50s). Both sets of our parents are still alive – mine are 80, and his are 92 and 86 – so genetically we "could" live fairly long lives. We want those lives to be as healthy as possible.

So far, we have both lost weight (16lb for me and 12lb for him) and find the fast days fairly easy. And we have both found that we do not overeat on the other days. In fact, I bought a four-finger Kit-Kat for the first time in months yesterday, ate only one finger and put the rest in my bag for later – absolutely unheard of for me as I have struggled with a very "healthy" appetite and have had an unhealthy BMI measurement for most of my life.

We have not had our IGF-1 measured, but we are both on high blood pressure medication, and my husband is on high-cholesterol medication. We are hopeful that we will see an improvement in these conditions when we next visit our GPs.

I actually find this way of eating much easier than any "diet" I have tried before. I can move the fast days around to cope with our social life.

As an update, I have now lost 20lb and am still finding the whole way of eating easy to do. On our fast days, we generally have a cooked breakfast (eggs or porridge) and then in the early evening a vegetable-heavy salad in the summer, or vegetable soup in the winter. My husband generally has a slice of bread as his extra 100 cals. We have maintained this way of eating since we saw the original programme and expect to continue (possibly with an interruption for Christmas).'

Maureen Johnston

'Thank you, Michael, for bringing this leading-edge science to our attention... We now feel in control of our health and weight for the first time in many years, and I'm committed to continuing the programme for life.'

Brian M

'Not shy about age size weight etc. I only really had a little to lose in comparision to some people so the health benefits are where I was most interest (I lost my Mum to breast cancer at 14 so the cancer avoiding benefits are something that appealed).

I am 38, but with every year that passed, I was getting heavier so weighing in at 10st 4lb on 01 Jan 2012 I pledged a plan of 'eat less, move more' – determined to lose some weight. A shoulder injury curtailed the 'move more' element, and my swimming and squash routine dried up but in August I watched a television programme that changed my attitude forever. Dr Moseley, (in his unique human guinea pig style) introduced me to ADF and 5:2 lifestyles and with the support of facebook groups and personal research I have stuck to an alternate day diet ever since.

At 5ft 2ins I wanted to get to mid 8stone 6lbs by 2013. The hardest part about regular dieting was combining eating times and portions with my family. The option of fasting means I skip out breakfast and lunch and eat a normal portion of healthy food at dinner time. The first few weeks were hard; trying to keep hydrated was tricky; but the most curious thing was my initial reaction in the first few days. I consider myself to have a healthy attitude to food and so I was alarmed at the mild panic I experienced on my first week of fasting. 'I cannot eat!' Once I realised I wasn't going to die and my energy levels didn't crash I began to relax, enjoy and now even look forward to my fast days.

Some of my best gym sessions are on restricted days; and the absence of food really has helped clear my mind, and improve my focus. And as for weight-loss: I am sure I am single handedly keeping the UK retail economy going. I have bought the same little black dress in three different sizes, as the weight has dropped off, I have bought a whole new gym wardrobe, and am loving the positive comments I am getting.

I am now evangelising about this to all friends and colleagues at work; some who are very sceptical and usually start with the response "Oooo, I couldn't last all day without food". But trust me – really, you can, and when you do realise how simple it is – it gets easier and easier. My mantra to my friends is: "you only diet for a day".

And the best bit: I really can eat all my favourite foods – pizza, curry, cheese, wine without gaining weight or feeling guilty. It's a lifestyle for me now, which means I will never need to diet again.]

Tara McLaughlin

‎ I've followed the 5:2 diet ever since watching Michael Mosley's TV programme. Its radically changed my attitude to food/hunger. I feel more energetic, and losing nearly a stone has been a delightful plus. I'm not the sort of person to follow "reducing" diets. It was the science that interested me. I know an amazing number of other people who also wouldn't "diet", but who are Intermittent Fasting. I actually value the fasting days in a way I never thought I would, which makes them easy to stick to. I don't intend to ever drop it.

Susie White

TWEETS

'Thank you for changing my lifestyle. Converted a bunch of people to ADF/5:2 thanks to u and @feedfastfeast FB group'
@Stickypippa

'As for me, have been IFasting since yr programme, changed my attitude to food/hunger, feel energetic & lost nearly a stone'
@cottagegardener

'After 4 months on 5:2, agree with your doc assessment... This could change the world. Your book should fuel the revolution.'
@alert_bri

'Overheard mums in playground today talking about you + 5:2. It's really catching on! Pleased as I've been doing it for ages.'
@alicia1980

'Thanks! We found the show very inspirational and from what people have tweeted us, lots of others did too. Love your shows'
@ValarWellbeing

CALORIE COUNTER

FOOD/PRODUCT	SERVING SIZE	KCALS
FRESH VEG		
Artichoke (globe)	100G	24
Artichoke (jerusalem)	100G	73
Arugula	100G	24
Asparagus	100G	27
Aubergine	100G	18
Avocado	100G	193
Beansprouts	100G	32
Beetroot	100G	38
Bell pepper	100G	30
Bok choy	100G	15
Broccoli	100G	32
Brussel sprouts	100G	43
Cabbage	100G	29
Carrot	100G	34
Cauliflower	100G	35
Celeriac	100G	17
Celery	100G	8
Chard	100G	17
Chickpea	100G	320
Chicory	100G	19
Collard greens	100G	33
Corn	100G	115
Courgette	100G	18
Closed cup mushrooms	100G	16

All values are raw product unless otherwise stated,
cereals are dried values unless otherwise stated

FOOD/PRODUCT	SERVING SIZE	KCALS
Cucumber	100G	10
Endive	100G	17
Fennel	100G	14
Floridix supplement	100ML	80
Frisée lettuce	100G	18
Garlic	100G	106
Green beans	100G	25
Iceberg lettuce	100G	14
Kale	100G	33
Leek	100G	23
Lentil	100G	319
Lettuce	100G	15
Mustard greens	100G	26
Onion (red)	100G	38
Onion (white)	100G	38
Peas, garden (frozen)	100G	86
Peas, petit pois	100G	52
Portobello mushrooms	100G	13
Potato (white)	100G	79
Radicchio	100G	19
Radish	100G	13
Rocket lettuce	100G	24
Romaine lettuce	100G	16
Round lettuce	100G	15
Samphire	100G	26
Shiitake mushrooms	100G	27
Spinach	100G	25
Squash	100G	40
Sweet potatoes	100G	93

FOOD/PRODUCT	SERVING SIZE	KCALS
Swiss chard	100G	19
Tomato	100G	20
Turnip	100G	24
Vitamin C tablets	100ML	2
Watercress	100G	26
Wheatgrass (frozen juice)	100G	17
FRUIT		
Açai (dried berry powder)	1G	5
Aloe	100G	3
Apples	100G	51
Apricots	100G	32
Bananas	100G	103
Black olives (pitted,drained)	100G	154
Blackberries	100G	26
Blueberries	100G	60
Cherries	100G	52
Cherries (glacé)	100G	313
Clementines	100G	41
Compote (apple & blackberry)	100G	107
Cranberries	100G	42
Dried apple	100G	310
Dried apricot	100G	196
Dried banana chips	100G	523
Dried blueberries	100G	313
Dried cranberries	100G	346
Dried dates (pitted)	100G	303
Dried figs	100G	229
Dried mango	100G	268

FOOD/PRODUCT	SERVING SIZE	KCALS
Dried prunes	100G	151
Figs	100G	230
Goji berries	100G	313
Grapefruit	100G	30
Grapes	100G	66
Kiwi	100G	55
Lemon	100G	20
Limes	100G	12
Mandarin	100G	35
Melon	100G	29
Nectarines	100G	44
Oranges	100G	40
Papaya	100G	40
Peaches	100G	37
Peaches (tinned)	100G	50
Pears	100G	41
Pears (tinned)	100G	37
Pineapple	100G	43
Pineapple (tinned)	100G	50
Plums	100G	39
Pomegranate	100G	55
Pomelo	100G	34
Prunes (tinned)	100G	90
Raisins	100G	292
Raspberries	100G	30
Satsumas	100G	31
Smoothies (strawberry/banana)	100ML	51
Strawberries	100G	28
Tangerines	100G	39

FOOD/PRODUCT	SERVING SIZE	KCALS
Watermelon	100G	33
HERBS AND SPICES		
Basil	1G	0
Cinnamon	1G	3
Cloves	1G	3
Coriander	1G	0
Cumin	1G	4
Ginger	1G	1
Lemongrass	1G	1
Mint	1G	0
Nutmeg	1G	4
Oregano	1G	3
Paprika	1G	3
Parsley	1G	0
Pepper	1G	3
Rosemary	1G	0
Saffron	1G	3
Sage	1G	3
Tamarind paste	100G	142
Tarragon	1G	0
Thyme	1G	2
Turmeric	1G	3
Vanilla pods	1G	3
OILS/FATS		
Butter (unsalted)	100G	739
Butter (salted)	100G	739
Canola oil	100ML	825

FOOD/PRODUCT	SERVING SIZE	KCALS
Corn oil	100ML	829
Hemp oil	100ML	837
Flaxseed oil	100ML	813
Lard	100G	899
Margarine	100G	735
Olive oil	100ML	823
Olive oil spread	100G	543
Rapeseed oil	100ML	825
Sunflower oil	100ML	828
Vegetable oil	100ML	827
Flora	100G	410
GRAINS		
Amaranth, grain	100G	368
Arborio rice	100G	354
Barley	100G	364
Basmati rice	100G	353
Bread (rye)	100G	242
Bread (spelt)	100G	241
Bread (pumpernickel)	100G	183
Bread (baguette)	100G	242
Bread (ciabatta)	100G	269
Bread (sourdough)	100G	256
Bread (soda, brown)	100G	223
Bread (pitta, white)	100G	265
Bread (chapati)	100G	278
Brown rice	100G	340
Buckwheat	100G	343
Buckwheat noodles	100G	363

FOOD/PRODUCT	SERVING SIZE	KCALS
Bulgar	100G	334
Corn (popping)	100G	339
Cous cous	100G	358
Cream crackers	100G	437
Gluten-free bread	100G	282
Granola	100G	432
Jasmine rice	100G	352
Long grain rice	100G	355
Matzo crackers	100G	381
Millet	100G	354
Muesli (unsweetened)	100G	353
Noodles (instant)	100G	450
Oats	100G	369
Oat cakes	100G	440
Oatmeal	100G	363
Porridge (ready to eat)	100G	95
Quinoa	100G	375
Ramen noodles	100G	361
Rice cakes	100G	379
Rice noodles	100G	373
Rye	100G	331
Rye bread	100G	242
Short grain rice	100G	351
Spelt	100G	314
Spelt bread	100G	241
Tortilla	100G	307
Triticale	100G	338
Udon noodles	100G	352
Vermicelli noodles	100G	354

FOOD/PRODUCT	SERVING SIZE	KCALS
Wheat berries	100G	326
Whole grain breads	100G	260
Whole grain cereal	100G	345
Whole grain pasta	100G	326
Whole wheat breads	100G	234
Whole wheat cereal	100G	359
Whole wheat pasta	100G	326
White rice	100G	355
Wild rice	100G	353
All bran	100G	334
Alpen	100G	361
Dorset cereal muesli	100G	356
Kallo milk choc rice cakes	100G	495
Quaker Oat So Simple instant porridge	100G	380
Ryvita (original)	100G	350
Special K	100G	379
Uncle Ben's white rice (long grain)	100G	344
PROTEIN		
Almonds (whole)	100G	613
Almonds (flaked)	100G	641
Almond (ground)	100G	618
Bacon	100G	244
Baked beans	100G	83
Beef, lean	100G	116
Black beans	100G	341
Burger (lamb)	100G	267
Burger (beef)	100G	283
Butter beans	100G	270

FOOD/PRODUCT	SERVING SIZE	KCALS
Cashews	100G	583
Calamari (battered, frozen)	100G	200
Chia seeds	100G	422
Chicken breast, skinless	100G	105
Chicken thigh, skinless	100G	163
Chickpeas	100G	320
Chipolata sausage	100G	267
Chorizo sausage	100G	348
Cod	100G	80
Dover sole	100G	78
Duck breast, skinless	100G	92
Edamame	100G	117
Egg whites	100G	50
Eggs (fried)	100G	187
Eggs (omelette)	100G	173
Eggs (poached)	100G	145
Eggs (scrambled)	100G	155
Fish, unbreaded	100G	76
Flageolet beans	100G	279
Flaxseed	100G	495
Garbanzo beans	100G	320
Goose	100G	356
Guinea fowl	100G	158
Haddock (fillets)	100G	74
Halibut	100G	100
Ham, lean	100G	104
Ham (pre-packaged, sliced)	100G	118
Hazelnuts	100G	660
Hemp seeds	100G	437

FOOD/PRODUCT	SERVING SIZE	KCALS
Hummus	100G	303
Lamb chops	100G	260
Lamb loin	100G	231
Lamb sausages	100G	260
Liver (chicken)	100G	122
Kidney beans	100G	311
Lima butter beans	100G	282
Lentils (red)	100G	327
Lentils (green)	100G	316
Lentils (yellow)	100G	334
Lentils (brown)	100G	297
Mackerel (fillets)	100G	204
Minced beef	100G	184
Minced lamb	100G	235
Minced pork	100G	140
Miso (paste)	100G	131
Mussels	100G	92
Navy beans	100G	285
Nuts (mixed, unsalted)	100G	661
Pâté	100G	322
Peanut butter, natural	100G	621
Peanuts	100G	561
Pinto beans	100G	309
Pistachio	100G	584
Pork, lean	100G	117
Pork sausage	100G	272
Prawns (King)	100G	69
Pumpkin seeds	100G	590
Rabbit	100G	137

FOOD/PRODUCT	SERVING SIZE	KCALS
Salami	100G	352
Salmon (canned)	100G	131
Salmon (fresh)	100G	215
Sardines (fresh)	100G	165
Sardines (tinned, in water)	100G	179
Sashimi	100G	137
Scallops	100G	83
Sea bass (fillets)	100G	133
Seafood (unbreaded)	100G	76
Sesame seeds	100G	616
Shrimp	100G	65
Soybeans	100G	375
Stewing beef	100G	121
Stewing lamb	100G	175
Sunflower seeds	100G	591
Sushi	100G	156
Tahini	100G	658
Tempeh	100G	172
Tofu	100G	70
Tuna (canned)	100G	108
Tuna (fresh)	100G	137
Turkey, skinless	100G	103
Veggie burgers	100G	137
Walnuts	100G	693
White beans	100G	285
White fish (steamed)	100G	83
Wild game, skinless (venison)	100G	101
Quorn (chicke-style pieces)	100G	114

FOOD/PRODUCT	SERVING SIZE	KCALS
DAIRY		
Almond milk	100ML	24
Cheddar cheese (low-fat)	100G	263
Cottage cheese (low-fat)	100G	72
Cow's milk cheese, Cheddar	100G	410
Cream cheese (low-fat)	100G	109
Crème fraiche (normal)	100ML	299
Crème fraiche (low-fat)	100ML	79
Custard	100G	118
Feta cheese	100G	276
Fromage frais	100G	105
Fruit yoghurt	100G	94
Goat cheese, soft	100G	324
Goat milk (whole)	100ML	61
Greek yoghurt	100G	132
Milk (whole)	100ML	64
Milk (semi skimmed)	100ML	50
Milk (1%)	100ML	41
Milk (skim)	100ML	35
Parmesan cheese (fresh, grated)	100G	389
Parmesan cheese (previously grated)	100G	389
Rice milk	100ML	46
Roquefort	100G	368
Ricotta	100G	134
Sour cream (normal)	100ML	192
Sour cream (low-fat)	100ML	104
Soy milk	100ML	42
Yoghurt (low-fat, with active cultures)	100G	66
Philadelphia cream cheese (normal)	100G	245

FOOD/PRODUCT	SERVING SIZE	KCALS
Philadelphia cream cheese (low-fat)	100G	111
SAUCES/DIPS/DRESSINGS		
Agave syrup	100G	296
Aioli	100G	611
Béarnaise sauce	100G	580
Barbecue sauce	100G	144
Bolognaise sauce (no meat)	100G	50
Capers	100G	32
Caramel sauce	100G	389
Chocolate sauce	100G	367
Chutney, tomato	100G	141
Coconut flakes	100G	632
Cornichons	100G	34
Cranberry sauce	100G	192
Gherkins	100G	38
Gravy (beef, readymade)	100G	45
Hollandaise sauce	100G	239
Honey	100G	334
Hummus	100G	303
Icing	100G	405
Jalapeño	100G	18
Jam (strawberry)	100G	258
Maple syrup	100G	265
Marmalade	100G	266
Mayonnaise (low-fat)	100ML	93
Mustard (dijon)	100G	160
Mustard (english)	100G	167
Mustard (grain)	100G	159

FOOD/PRODUCT	SERVING SIZE	KCALS
Nutella	100G	529
Pesto	100G	431
Piccalili sauce	100G	80
Pickled onions	100G	36
Pickles	100G	20
Roasted aubergine spread/dip	100G	102
Roasted red pepper spread/dip	100G	235
Salad dressing (balsamic)	100ML	209
Salad dressing (caesar no fat)	100ML	61
Salad dressing (olive oil and lemon)	100ML	439
Salad dresssing (low-calorie)	100ML	58
Salsa	100G	68
Soy sauce	100ML	105
Spirulina, powder	100G	374
Sriracha	100ML	98
Sundried tomatoes	100G	167
Taramasalata	100G	516
Tartare sauce	100G	358
Tomato and basil sauce	100G	60
Tomato ketchup	100G	102
Tikka masala sauce	100G	133
Treacle	100G	294
Tzatzkiki	100G	137
Vegemite	100G	189
Vinegar (balsamic)	100ML	138
Vinegar (red wine)	100ML	23
Vinegar (white wine)	100ML	22
Whipped cream	100ML	368
Heinz salad cream	100G	333

FOOD/PRODUCT	SERVING SIZE	KCALS
HP brown sauce	100G	119
Lea & Perrins	100ML	115
Marmite	100G	252
DRINKS		
Apple juice	100ML	44
Beer, bitter	100ML	32
Beer, lager	100ML	43
Cappuccino, whole milk	100ML	37
Capuccino, skimmed milk	100ML	22
Champagne	100ML	76
Coffee (black)	100ML	0
Coffee (with semi-sk milk)	100ML	7
Cordial (lime)	100ML	24
Cordial (elderflower)	100ML	27
Espresso	100ML	20
Gin and tonic	100ML	70
Ginger ale (dry)	100ML	34
Hot chocolate	100ML	59
Hot chocolate (low-cal)	100ML	19
Hot milk and honey (semi-sk)	100ML	58
Latte (whole milk)	100ML	54
Latte (skimmed milk)	100ML	29
Lemonade	100ML	47
Lime juice	100ML	23
Macchiato (whole milk)	100ML	30
Macchiato (skimmed milk)	100ML	26
Milkshakes (strawberry)	100ML	67
Orange juice	100ML	42

FOOD/PRODUCT	SERVING SIZE	KCALS
Orange squash	100ML	10
Pear juice	100ML	43
Red wine	100ML	68
Sparkling water	100ML	0
Tea (black)	100ML	0
Tea (chai latte, semi-sk)	100ML	70
Tea (green)	100ML	0
Tea (herbal)	100ML	0
Vodka tonic	100ML	71
White wine	100ML	66
Sprite	100ML	44
Coca cola	100ML	43
Coke (diet)	100ML	0
Coke (normal)	100ML	43
Innocent smoothy (strawberry/banana)	100ML	53
Innocent smoothy (mango)	100ML	56
Ribena	100ML	43
SANDWICHES		
Ham and cheese	100G	288
Egg and cress	100G	232
Cheese and chutney	100G	228
Tuna salad	100G	221
SOUPS		
Bouillon	100ML	7
Carrot and coriander	100G	35
Chicken noodle	100G	35
Chowder	100G	53

FOOD/PRODUCT	SERVING SIZE	KCALS
Leek and potato	100G	53
Light broth	100G	36
Lobster bisque	100G	68
Miso	100G	22
Onion	100G	45
Passata	100G	31
Pho (beef with noodles)	100G	66
Tomato and basil	100G	40
Vegetable	100G	45
Heinz cream of mushroom	100G	50
Heinz tomato	100G	59
CAKES/BISCUITS/DESSERTS		
Apple pie	100G	262
Apple tart	100G	265
Baklava	100G	498
Brownies	100G	419
Carrot cake, iced	100G	359
Chewing gum, sugarfree	100G	159
Chocolate (dark)	100G	547
Chocolate (milk)	100G	549
Chocolate (white)	100G	567
Chocolate cake, iced	100G	414
Chocolate chip cookies	100G	499
Chocolate-covered raisins	100G	418
Cinnamon buns	100G	280
Chocolate mousse	100G	174
Chocolate croissant	100G	433
Crystallized ginger	100G	351

FOOD/PRODUCT	SERVING SIZE	KCALS
Ice cream, vanilla	100G	190
Flapjacks, all-butter	100G	457
Lemon cake	100G	366
Liquorice	100G	325
Marshmallow	100G	338
Meringue	100G	394
Mince pies	100G	398
Oatmeal raisin cookies	100G	445
Pain aux raisins	100G	335
Peppermints	100G	395
Scones	100G	366
Sherbert, lemon	100G	390
Shortbread, all-butter	100G	523
Sorbet, lemon	100G	118
Tiramisu	100G	263
Toffee	100G	459
Yoghurt-covered dried fruit	100G	447
Cadbury's dairy milk	100G	525
Haribo	100G	344
Digestives – Mcvities	100G	478
Green and Black's 70% chocolate	100G	575
Green and Black's 85% chocolate	100G	630
Hob Nobs – Mcvities	100G	473
Jaffa cakes	100G	377
Lindt 70% chocolate	100G	540
Tic tacs	100G	391
Wine gums	100G	325

FOOD/PRODUCT	SERVING SIZE	KCALS
SAVOURY SNACKS		
Bagels	100G	256
Breadsticks	100G	408
Cheese straws	100G	520
Crumpets	100G	180
French fries (oven-baked)	100G	260
Meat pies	100G	293
Muffins (blueberry)	100G	387
Pizza (Margherita)	100G	258
Plain croissant	100G	414
Popcorn (salty)	100G	520
Popcorn (sweet)	100G	493
Potato chips (readysalted)	100G	529
Quiche Lorraine	100G	261
Peanuts (unsalted)	100G	561
Salted peanuts	100G	621
Salted mixed nuts	100G	667
Samosas (vegetable)	100G	225
Sausage roll	100G	340
Vegetable chips	100G	502

Data provided by www.nutracheck.co.uk

ENDNOTES AND RESEARCH PAPERS

[1]Barry M Popkin; Kiyah J Duffey. 'Does hunger and satiety drive eating anymore? Increasing eating occasions and decreasing time between eating occasions in the United States'. *American Journal of Clinical Nutrition*, May 2010

[2]Mark Mattson; Edward Calabrese. 'When a little poison is good for you', *New Scientist* magazine, 06 August 2008

[3]Carlson AJ; Hoelzel, F. Department of Physiology, University of Chicago, US. 'Apparent prolongation of the life span of rats by intermittent fasting'. *Journal of Nutrition*, 1945. www.jn.nutrition.org/content/31/3/363.full.pdf

[4]Bergamini E, Cavallini G, Donati A, Gori Z, Pisa, Italy. 'The role of autophagy in aging: its essential part in the anti-aging mechanism of caloric restriction'. *Annals of the New York Academy of Science,* October 2007

[5]Varady, KA; Surabhi Bhutani; Church EC; Kempel, M. 'Short-term modified alternate-day fasting: a novel dietary strategy for weight loss and cardio-protection in obese adults.'. *American Journal of Clinical Nutrition*, November 2009
&
Klempel MC, Kroeger CM, Varady KA. 'Alternate day fasting (ADF) with a high-fat diet produces similar weight loss and cardio-protection as ADF with a low-fat diet.' *Metabolism.* January 2013; 62(1):137-43

[6]M N Harvie et al. Genesis Prevention Centre, University Hospital of South Manchester NHS Foundation Trust, UK. 'Intermittent, low-carbohydrate diets more successful than standard dieting; possible intervention for breast cancer prevention'. Presentation at the CTRC-AACR San Antonio Breast Cancer Symposium, December 2011. www.aacr.org/home/public--media/aacr-press-releases.aspx?d=2649

[7]Hatori, M; Vollmers, C; Zarrinpar, A; DiTacchio, L et al. Salk

Institute for Biological Studies, La Jolla, CA, US. 'Time-Restricted Feeding without Reducing Caloric Intake Prevents Metabolic Diseases in Mice Fed a High-Fat Diet'. *Cell Metabolism*, 2012

[8]Erickson, KI; Voss, MW, et al. Salk Institute, San Diego, CA, US. 'Exercise training increases size of hippocampus and improves memory'. *Proceedings of the National Academy of Science USA*, January, 2011

[9]Halagappa VK, Guo Z, Pearson M, Matsuoka Y, Cutler RG, Laferla FM, Mattson MP, National Institute on Ageing, Baltimore, MD, US. 'Intermittent fasting and caloric restriction ameliorate age-related behavioral deficits in the triple-transgenic mouse model of Alzheimer's disease'. *Neurobiology of Disease*, April 2007

[10]Shirayama Y, Chen AC, Nakagawa S, Russell DS, Duman RS. ale University School of Medicine, New Haven, Connecticut, US. 'Brain-derived neurotrophic factor produces antidepressant effects in behavioral models of depression'. *Journal of Neuroscience*, April 2002

[11]Li B, Suemaru K, Kitamura Y, Cui R, Gomita Y, Araki H. Department of Clinical Pharmacology and Pharmacy, Brain Science, Ehime University Hospital, Japan. 'Strategy to develop a new drug for treatment-resistant depression--role of electroconvulsive stimuli and BDNF'. *Yakugaku Zasshi*, April 2007

[12]Nils Halberg, Morten Henriksen, Nathalie Söderhamn, Bente Stallknecht, Thorkil Ploug, Peter Schjerling and Flemming Dela. Department of Muscle Research Centre, The Panum Institute, University of Copenhagen, Denmark. 'Effect of intermittent fasting and refeeding on insulin action in healthy men'. *Journal of Applied Physiology*, December 2005

[13]Raffaghello L, Lee C, Safdie FM, Wei M, Madia F, Bianchi G, Longo VD. Andrus Gerontology Center, Department of Biological Sciences and Norris Cancer Center, University of Southern California, LA, CA, US. 'Starvation-dependent differential stress resistance protects normal but not cancer cells against high-dose chemotherapy'. *Proceedings of the National Academy of sciences of the United States of America*, June 2008

[14]Lee C; Longo V et al. University of Southern California. 'FastingCycles Retard Growth of Tumours and Sensitize a Range of Cancer Cell Types to Chemotherapy'. *Science Translational Medicine*, Feb 2012.

[15]Safdie F; Dorff T; Longo V et al. University of Southern California. 'Fasting and Cancer Treatment in Humans', *Aging* 2009

[16]Stradling JR, Crosby JH. Osler Chest Unit, Churchill Hospital, Oxford. 'Predictors and prevalence of obstructive sleep apnoea and snoring in 1001 middle aged men'. *Thorax*, February 1991

[17]Michelle N. Harvie et al. Genesis Prevention Centre, University Hospital of South Manchester NHS Foundation Trust, UK. 'The effects of intermittent or continuous energy restriction on weight loss and metabolic disease risk markers: a randomised trial in young overweight women' *International Journal of Obesity* (London), May 2011

[18]Leidy HJ; Tang M; Armstrong C; Martin CB; Campbell WW. University of Missouri, US. 'The Effects of Consuming Frequent, Higher Protein Meals on Appetite and Satiety During Weight Loss in Overweight/Obese Men.' *Obesity* 2011
&
Astrup, A. Department of Human Nutrition, Centre for Advanced Food Studies, Royal Veterinary and Agricultural University, Copenhagen, Denmark. 'The satiating power of protein – a key to obesity prevention?' *American Society for Clinical Nutrition*, July 2005
&
Halton, T; Hu, F. Department of Nutrition, Harvard School of Public Health, Boston MA, US. 'The Effects of High Protein Diets on Thermogenesis, Satiety and Weight Loss'. *Journal of the American College of Nutrition*, October 2004

[19]Cara B. Ebbeling, David S. Ludwig et al, New Balance Foundation Obesity Prevention Center, Boston, Massachusetts, US. 'Effects of Dietary Composition on Energy Expenditure During Weight-Loss Maintenance'. *Journal of the American Medical Association*, June 2012

[20]O'Neil, C; Nicklas T. Louisiana State University Agricultural

Center, Baton Rouge, Louisiana. 'Nut Consumption Is Associated with Decreased Health Risk Factors for Cardiovascular Disease and Metabolic Syndrome in U.S. Adults'. *Journal of the American College of Nutrition*, December 2011
&
Ros, E; Tapsell LC; Sabate J. Lipid Clinic, Endocrinology and Nutrition Service, Institut d'Investigacions Biomèdiques August Pi i Sunyer, Hospital Clínic, Barcelona, Spain. 'Nuts and berries for heart health'. *Current Atherosclerosis Reports*, November 2010

[21]Dhurandhar N. Pennington Biomedical Research Center, Louisiana, US. 'Egg Proteins For Breakfast Keeps You Feeling Full For Longer'

[22]*Mindless Eating – Why We Eat More Than We Think*, by Brian Wansink (Bantam-Dell 2006)

[23]Mann, T; Tomiyama, A. J; Westling, E; Lew, A; Samuels, B; Chatman, J. UCLA. 'Medicare's search for effective obesity treatments: Diets are not the answer'. *American Psychologist*, April 2007

[24]www.marksdailyapple.com/health-benefits-of-intermittent-fasting/#axzz2DQjnYyUz

[25]Dom Joly, *The Independent*, November 11, 2012. www.independent.co.uk/voices/comment/ive-discovered-how-to-lose-weight-fast-8303657.html

[26]Van Proeyen K, Szlufcik K, Nielens H, Pelgrim K, Deldicque L, Hesselink M, Van Veldhoven PP, Hespel P. Research Centre for Exercise and Health, Department of Biomedical Kinesiology, Leuven, Belgium. 'Training in the fasted state improves glucose tolerance during fat-rich diet'. Journal of Physiology, November 2010

[27]Morewedge CK, Young Eun Huh, and Vosgerau J. Carnegie Mellon University, Pittsburgh, PA, USA. 'Thought for Food: Imagined Consumption Reduces Actual Consumption'. *Science*, December 2010

[28]Huff, MW. Robarts. Research Institute at the University of Western Ontario, Canada. 'Nobiletin Attenuates VLDL Overproduction, Dyslipidemia, and Atherosclerosis in Mice With Diet-Induced Insulin

Resistance'. *American Journal of Diabetes*, May 2011

[29]Mulvihill EE; Alister EM; Sutherland BG; Telford DE; Sawyer CG; Edwards JY; Markle JM; Hegele RA; Huff MW. Robarts Research Institute at the University of Western Ontario, Canada. 'Naringenin prevents dyslipidemia, apoB overproduction and hyperinsulinemia in LDL-receptor null mice with diet-induced insulin resistance'. *Diabetes*, 2009

[30]Fujioka K; Greenway F; Sheard J; Ying Y. Scripps Clinic, La Jolla, California, US. 'The effects of grapefruit on weight and insulin resistance: relationship to the metabolic syndrome'. *Journal of Medicinal Food*, 2006

[31]Schrenk D. Geisenheim Research Center, Germany. 'Pectin, Fat Absorption and Anti-Carcinogenic Effects'. *Nutrition*, April 2008

[32]A. Venket Rao; Sanjiv Agarwal, Department of Nutritional Sciences, Faculty of Medicine, University of Toronto, Canada. 'Role of Antioxidant Lycopene in Cancer and Heart Disease'. *Journal of the American College of Nutrition*, October 2000

[33]Jouni Karppi; Jari A. Laukkanen; Juhani Sivenius; Kimmo Ronkainen; Sudhir Kurl. Department of Medicine, Institute of Public Health and Clinical Nutrition, University of Eastern Finland, Kuopio. 'Serum lycopene decreases the risk of stroke in men'. *Neurology*, October 2012

[34]Moghe, S. Texas Woman's University, Denton, Texas, US. 'Blueberries may inhibit development of fat cells'. Federation of American Societies for Experimental Biology, *Science Daily*, April 2011

[35]Talia Miron; Irina Shin; Guy Feigenblat; Lev Weiner; David Mirelman; Meir Wilchek; Aharon Rabinkov. Department of Biological Chemistry, The Weizmann Institute of Science, Rehovot, Israel. 'A spectrophotometric assay for allicin, alliin, and alliinase'. *Analytical Biochemistry*, 2002

[36]Rolls B; Flood J. Penn State University US. 'Eating Soup Will Help Cut Calories at Meals', presented at the Experimental Biology

Conference in Washington, May 2007

[37]Rui Hai Liu. Department of Food Science, Cornell University, New York, US. 'Thermal Processing Enhances the Nutritional Value of Tomatoes by Increasing Total Antioxidant Activity'. *Journal of Agricultural and Food Chemistry*, April 2002

[38]Miglio, C; Chiavaro, E; Visconti A; Fogliano V. Department of Public Health, University of Parma, Italy. 'Effects of Different Cooking Methods on Nutritional and Physicochemical Characteristics of Selected Vegetables'. *Journal of Agricultural and Food Chemistry*, December 2007

[39]Herman CP, Mack D. 'Restrained and unrestrained eating'. *Journal of Personality*, 1975

[40]Schusdziarra V; Hausmann M; Wittke C; Mittermeier J; Kellner M; Naumann A; Wagenpfeil S; Erdmann J. University of Munich (2011). 'Impact of breakfast on daily energy intake – an analysis of absolute versus relative breakfast calories'. *Nutrition Journal*, January 2011

[41]Mesas AE; Leon-Munoz LM; Lopez-Garcia E. Department of Preventive Medicine and Public Health, School of Medicine, Universidad Autónoma de Madrid, Spain. 'The effect of coffee on blood pressure and cardiovascular disease in hypertensive individuals'. *American Journal of Clinical Nutrition*, 2011
&
Larsson S; Orsini N. National Institute of Environmental Medicine, Karolinska Institutet, Stockholm, Sweden. 'Coffee Consumption and Risk of Stroke: A Dose-Response Meta-Analysis of Prospective Studies'. *American Journal of Epidemiology*, September 2011
&
Anna Floegel, Tobias Pischon, Manuela M Bergmann, Birgit Teucher, Rudolf Kaaks, Heiner Boeing. European Prospective Investigation into Cancer and Nutrition (EPIC), Germany. 'Coffee consumption and risk of chronic disease' *American Society for Nutrition*, April 2012

[42]Kirkendall DT, Leiper JB, Bartagi Z, Dvorak J, Zerguini Y. FIFA Medical Assessment and Research Centre, Schulthess Clinic, Zurich, Switzerland . 'The influence of Ramadan on physical performance

measures in young Muslim footballers'. *Journal of Sports Science,* December 2008

[43]Van Proeyen K, Szlufcik K, Nielens H, Ramaekers M, Hespel P. Research Centre for Exercise and Health, Department of Biomedical Kinesiology, Leuven, Belgium. 'Beneficial metabolic adaptations due to endurance exercise training in the fasted state'. *Journal of Applied Physiology,* January 2011

[44]Harber MP, Konopka AR, Jemiolo B, Trappe SW, Trappe TA, Reidy PT. Human Performance Laboratory, Ball State University, Muncie, IN, US. 'Muscle protein synthesis and gene expression during recovery from aerobic exercise in the fasted and fed states'. *American Journal of Physiology,* November 2010

[45]Deldicque L, De Bock K, Maris M, Ramaekers M, Nielens H, Francaux M, Hespel P. Department of Biomedical Kinesiology, Leuven, Belgium. 'Increased p70s6k phosphorylation during intake of a protein-carbohydrate drink following resistance exercise in the fasted state'. *European Journal of Applied Physiology,* March 2010

[46]Quote from www.marksdailyapple.com/fasting-exercise-workout-recovery/

[47]Van Proeyen K, Szlufcik K, Nielens H, Pelgrim K, Deldicque L, Hesselink M, Van Veldhoven PP, Hespel P. Research Centre for Exercise and Health, Department of Biomedical Kinesiology, Leuven, Belgium. 'Training in the fasted state improves glucose tolerance during fat-rich diet'. *Journal of Physiology,* November 2010

[48] *The New York Times,* September 15, 2010 www.well.blogs.nytimes.com/2010/12/15/phys-ed-the-benefits-of-exercising-before-breakfast/?src=me&ref=general

[49]Tarnopolsky, MA. McMaster University Medical Center, Hamilton, Ontario, Canada. 'Gender Differences in Substrate Metabolism During Endurance Exercise'. *Canadian Journal of Applied Physiology,* 2000

[50]Stannard SR, Buckley AJ, Edge JA, Thompson MW. Institute of Food Nutrition and Human Health, Massey University, New Zealand. 'Adaptations to skeletal muscle with endurance exercise training in the acutely fed versus overnight-fasted state'. *Journal of Science and Medicine in Sport*, July 2010

[51]Heilbronn LK, Smith SR, Martin CK, Anton SD, Ravussin E. Pennington Biomedical Research Center, Baton Rouge, LA, US. 'Alternate-day fasting in non-obese subjects: effects on body weight, body composition, and energy metabolism'. *American Journal of Clinical Nutrition*, January 2005

[52]Webber J, Macdonald IA. Department of Physiology and Pharmacology, University of Nottingham Medical School, UK. 'The cardiovascular, metabolic and hormonal changes accompanying acute starvation in men and women'. *British Journal of Nutrition*. March 1994

[53]Heilbronn LK, Smith SR, Martin CK, Anton SD, Ravussin E. Pennington Biomedical Research Center, Baton Rouge, LA, US. 'Alternate-day fasting in non-obese subjects: effects on body weight, body composition, and energy metabolism'. *American Journal of Clinical Nutrition*, January 2005

[54]Heilbronn LK, Smith SR, Martin CK, Anton SD, Ravussin E. Pennington Biomedical Research Center, Baton Rouge, LA, US. 'Alternate-day fasting in non-obese subjects: effects on body weight, body composition, and energy metabolism'. *American Journal of Clinical Nutrition*, January 2005

For further reading, we recommend Brad Pilon's e-book *Eat Stop Eat*, available from www.bradpilon.com, and www.marksdailyapple.com – a great resource for would-be fasters who want to learn more.

ACKNOWLEDGEMENTS

This book would not have been possible without the many scientists who gave so generously of their time and their research. They include Dr Luigi Fontana of Washington University School of Medicine; Professor Mark Mattson of the National Institute on Aging; Dr Krista Varady of the University of Illinois at Chicago; and Professor Valter Longo, director of the USC Longevity Institute.

A huge thanks to Aidan Laverty, editor of BBC's *Horizon*, who pointed me towards the brave new world of Intermittent Fasting, and to the entire production team, but especially Kate Dart and Roshan Samarasinghe. I'd also like to thank Janice Hadlow who was brave enough to first put me in front of the camera and gave me the chance to try new things.

Thank you to Nicola Jeal at *The Times* for her constant ingenuity and support.

Our thanks also go to Rebecca Nicolson, Aurea Carpenter and Emmie Francis at Short Books, for their hard work and immediate grasp of the Fast Diet's life-changing potential.

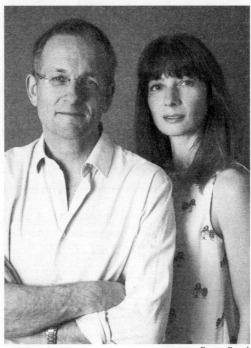
Romas Foord

AUTHOR BIOGS

Michael Mosley did a first degree at Oxford University before training to be a doctor at the Royal Free Hospital in London. After qualifying he joined the BBC, where he has been a science journalist, executive producer and, more recently, a well known television presenter. Unusually, he has written and presented series on BBC One, Two, Three and Four as well as BBC Radio Four. He has won numerous television awards, including an RTS (Royal Television Award) and being named Medical Journalist of the Year by the British Medical Association. He is married to a doctor and has four children, amongst them a son who is at medical school.

For more than 20 years, Mimi Spencer has written features for national newspapers and magazines in the UK, including *The Observer*, *The Times*, *Vogue* and *Harper's Bazaar*. As the Fashion Editor of the *London Evening Standard*, she won the British Fashion Journalist of the Year Award in 2000, and went on to edit the paper's weekly title, *ES Magazine*.

Mimi has had a column in *You Magazine* at the *Mail on Sunday* for over a decade. In 2009, drawing on her personal and career interest in women's attitudes to weight loss, she wrote *101 Things to do Before You Diet* (Doubleday/Rodale).

Today, she writes regularly on women's issues and lifestyle for the *Saturday Times*, *Marie Claire*, *Red* and other magazines. She lives in Brighton on the south coast of England with her husband, two children, a small boat and an endlessly hungry dog.

INDEX